THE OLDER PATIENT AND THE ROLE OF THE PHYSIOTHERAPIST

ff

THE OLDER PATIENT AND THE ROLE OF THE PHYSIOTHERAPIST

Margot Hawker MCSP, DipTP

with contributions from
D. Mandelstam MCSP, DipSocSc, J. Priest MCSP, DipTP,
A. Squires MCSP, J. Stephenson MCSP, P. Turnbull MCSP, DipPE

with a Foreword by Donald Dick MA(Cantab), MB, BChir, FRCPsych, DPM
Consultant Psychiatrist, Herrison Hospital, Dorset
formerly Director of the Health Advisory Service

faber and faber
LONDON · BOSTON

Originally published as *Geriatrics for Physiotherapists and the Allied Professions*, 1974
First published under this title 1985
by Faber and Faber Limited
3 Queen Square, London WC1N 3AU

Set by Goodfellow & Egan Typesetting Ltd, Cambridge
Printed in Great Britain by
Whitstable Litho Ltd, Whitstable, Kent

British Library Cataloguing in Publication Data

Hawker, Margaret
The older patient and the role of the physiotherapist.—2nd ed.
1. Geriatrics 2. Physical therapy
I. Title II. Hawker, Margaret. Geriatrics for physiotherapists and the allied professions
618.97 RC953.5

ISBN 0 571 13427 0

CONTENTS

FOREWORD

The thoughtful management of an ageing population is one of the most challenging problems for the health services of our time. It is not that people are living longer but that more and more are reaching old age in comparative good health. The old bear the scars of a lifetime, the harvest of past illnesses, former stresses and indulgences that did not seem to matter much at the time. As the vitality of organs fades towards the end of long life the ability to cope independently also fades. It is not, as Margot Hawker reminds us in an early chapter, that old age is an illness, it is a cumulation of the unique biography, the experiences and circumstances of an individual who is beginning to wind down biologically. To this is added what has happened to the body and mind of the individual over the years. The result is like a balance sheet of debts and credits with which to encounter the last age of all.

Our society strives that, in old age, its citizens should if possible have comfort, dignity and independence, with sufficient community, health and welfare services to meet their needs and to balance some of the debts, of the years. The key to independence and the enjoyment of activities, even of dignity, is very often mobility. Incontinence of urine can simply be the result of being unable to get up and go. Restricted movement may limit the ability to dress or enjoy pleasant activities outside the home. An old person may be well in every other respect but frustrated beyond endurance at not being able to manage simple personal tasks (who can preserve dignity while being helped on to a lavatory seat?). Now this is the point at which one begins to realise the importance of physiotherapists for the older patient. Many old people lead restricted lives, not because of the failures of medical treatment or wise nursing but because of unfinished rehabilitation. Because no one has sought to find a way round the restrictions imposed by disability. If medicine, nursing and the social services have done their best, is there nothing more? This is the challenge for physiotherapists: to become deeply involved in the work of clinical teams looking after elderly people, to contribute fully to team decisions and to widen the horizon to take in the whole lifestyle of the patient and the capacity for engagement. Physiotherapy for the older patient needs a very broad base. It needs an understanding of what ageing means in the modern world, the impact of illness in old age, a knowledge of the illnesses of old age, what is available for the elderly in the community, how old people get help or supplements to their income. Further it requires a knowledge of the services for old people in hospital, in their own homes and in residential care. It is on this base that the physiotherapist can build a contribution to the work common to all disciplines and make specialist use of the skills and techniques of physiotherapy. These skills are for sharing, and often the main contribution of a physiotherapist is to educate and sustain the work of other professionals in achieving the best deal for the patient.

In addressing these issues Margot Hawker has divided her book into two parts. The first part is an overview of services for old people, the second describes the role of the physiotherapist in the care of the elderly. She brings to both aspects a well-informed approach and a vast practical experience. In Part I she summarises current thinking on the problems of old age in our society and the services that are provided for the elderly. She illustrates with a selection of quotations from authorities in the field in the United Kingdom, with many of whom she has a working acquaintance. She draws upon her work with the Health Advisory Service and the experience of being asked to advise on the organisation of services in the NHS and voluntary bodies. It is in this part that attitudes and expectations are examined: that is, the context of physiotherapy in old age. If we are encouraged to practise 'whole person medicine' then why is whole person physiotherapy less of an aim?

The physiotherapist is invited to move out of the physiotherapy department for some of the time, retaining the professional skills of individual treatment but also seeing how they can apply in a wider context. Old people present a range of problems in some of which the physiotherapist is the principal therapist, in others she acts as contributor, adviser or supervisor. An understanding of the old person, preferably in his or her own habitat is clearly essential. How do the residual assets of function or personality fit in with the real world in which the old person lives? Who is available to help? Do the relatives need to be taught to be aides? Are there further improvements in function which might first tip the balance towards greater self-determination and dignity? Margot Hawker tackles the borders of her profession with vigour, seeking the place of physiotherapy among the other clinical disciplines. The importance of multidisciplinary teamwork is not just the warm bonhomie of working together with colleagues. It is also making certain that the set tasks of each separate discipline are known to the others and that their completion may depend upon the work of two or three disciplines working together. The ideal ward meeting allows each discipline to describe the residual problems of their special interest, plans the next moves and assesses progress in reaching the aims set at the previous meeting. Ultimately all tasks may be complete except those, say of the physiotherapist or social worker. It is at this stage that the principal decision about management passes to the discipline that still has tasks to complete.

In Part II, the practical involvement of the physiotherapist in the management of the elderly is described. Proper importance is given to the way that services should be organised. The sections on community physiotherapy and psychogeriatric services are especially welcome to those of us concerned with the aim of trying to manage the failing elderly in their own domestic surroundings. The impact of good physiotherapy services in units for the elderly mentally ill is becoming increasingly apparent. The intervention of physiotherapy often tips the balance between continued family management or independent management and admission to residential care. The growing interest of physiotherapists in the elderly mentally ill and indeed the community management of elderly people gives room for pioneering work for a group of enthusiasts. The sections on dressing and incontinence show the immense practical experience that Mrs Hawker brings to her book. The obvious grasp of the subject gained from doing, as well as thinking about the work validates the rest of the book.

What, therefore, are the lessons to be learned from this thoughtful book? It examines attitudes to services for the elderly and places them in context both for physiotherapists and in their links with each component service. It challenges physiotherapists to be out and about in the community, with other disciplines and to make service and practical contributions to the range of needs that old people present. It should much broaden the readers horizons.

Herrison Hospital
Dorchester, Dorset

Donald Dick, 1985

CONTRIBUTORS

Mrs Margot Hawker MCSP, DipTP
Formerly District Physiotherapist,
Edgware and Hendon Health Authority
Now Family Support Service Adviser
Leonard Cheshire Foundation, London

Mrs Dorothy Mandelstam MCSP, DipSocSc
Incontinence Adviser, Disabled Living Foundation
380–384 Harrow Road
London W9 2HU

Miss Jill Priest MCSP, DipTP
Superintendent Physiotherapist
Banstead Hospital
Sutton SM2 5PA

Mrs Amanda Squires MCSP
Superintendent Physiotherapist
St Francis' Hospital
London SE22 8DF

Miss Jennifer Stephenson MCSP
Superintendent Community Physiotherapist
St Mary Abbot's Hospital
London W8 3LQ

Mrs Peggy Turnbull MCSP, DipPE
Clothing Adviser, Disabled Living Foundation
380–384 Harrow Road
London W9 2HU

ACKNOWLEDGEMENTS

In writing this book, I am particularly indebted to the five physiotherapy contributors. In sharing their specialist knowledge, they have demonstrated some of the wide range of expertise required to meet the needs of elderly patients.

To Dr Donald Dick, formerly Director of the NHS Health Advisory Service, I want to extend my warm appreciation for accepting the invitation to write the Foreword.

Finally, a special word of thanks to Mrs Kay Bainbridge and Mrs Terry McArthy who have worked so unstintingly on the typing and retyping of the manuscript.

M.H., *1985*

INTRODUCTION

The immediate predecessor to this book, *Geriatrics for Physiotherapists and the Allied Professions*, was written mainly for therapists working in departments of geriatric medicine. The philosophy of geriatric medicine which involves total patient care and management, the provision of a comprehensive domiciliary and hospital-based service together with close collaboration with local statutory and voluntary agencies, has equal relevance today as it had when that book was published 10 years ago.

However, in the intervening time, the number of elderly people has continued to increase, both in terms of absolute numbers and as a percentage of the population as a whole. Today, the major proportion of disabled adults both at home and in hospital is over the age of 65.

The complex needs of older patients, particularly the very elderly, and the growing public expectations put increasing pressures on scarce remedial resources. No single profession can be expected to provide all the answers, but it should be possible for each individual physiotherapist to know where to obtain help, to be aware of what other disciplines can offer and to be prepared to find ways of working more closely with others concerned across departmental boundaries and between hospital and community in order to share knowledge and skills in the effective management of elderly people with disability.

In this book some of the needs of older people and the services provided for them are described against the wider backcloth of a society which is moving with ever-growing speed into an age of ageing with all that such demographic change implies.

Part One

AN OVERVIEW

Chapter One

AN AGEING SOCIETY

When is a person to be called old? To Pablo Casals at 93 age was a relative matter, for as he said, 'Each day I am reborn, each day I must begin again.' For him and many like him, life can be a continuing and expanding experience and although as in Casals' case people may be old in chronological terms, life for them will go on evolving, holding challenge, zest and increasing enrichment.

For others, old age is looked upon as one of a series of stages in life, perhaps in a less negative fashion than the view Shakespeare has bequeathed us, but still as a milestone that has to be checked off as we progress through the years. There can be pre-school groups, teenage groups, young wives or young marrieds, the over 35s, pre-retirement groups and the over 60s. Not only do such groupings oversimplify the whole situation since they tend to overlook the widespread individual differences between people at any age, but as Irene Gore says in her book *Age and Vitality* we build up anxieties about each stage in life before we enter it. 'We dread the Rubicons before we come to them . . . We need to be liberated from these dread milestones and to judge the quality of our life at any time on its own merits' (Gore, 1979).

There are two kinds of ageing. There is the biological process that happens to all of us and if, as we see later in this chapter, we live in an industrialised society, there is a very good chance that we shall go on living to the age of 70 and frequently a good deal longer.

The other concept of ageing is created by the society in which we live and the role that we, as a society, have imposed upon people as they reach retirement age. (In the United Kingdom the term elderly is used to cover all individuals at and above the minimum age at which the National Insurance retirement pension can be paid: currently for men at 65 years of age and for women at 60 – soon possibly to be telescoped to 63 for both sexes.) Retirement involves a radical change in the daily lives of people who have previously been in employment, and for many in our work-orientated society it is the beginning of a humiliating process leading to the slow erosion of confidence and personal self-esteem. As Alex Comfort (1977), one of the world's leading gerontologists says, 'Modern research indicates that a high proportion of the mental and attitudinal changes seen in "old people" are not biological effects of ageing. They are the result of role-playing . . . the part we assign "the old" is a destructive part. They are supposed to be physically and intellectually infirm, slow on the uptake and rigid in their ways.'

Gerontology is an academic subject concerned with characterising the normal ageing process in structural and fundamental terms. Its highest aim is to attempt to understand not only how, but why, people age. While it is relatively easy to characterise ageing in physical terms, the fundamental biological mechanisms which cause us to age are more difficult to probe and are as yet unknown.

WHAT IS AGEING?

Strictly speaking, the process of ageing starts with embryonic and fetal development. However, it is usual to regard ageing as the sum of those changes in structure and function which take place after reproductive maturity has been reached and which result first in a decreased adaptation of the individual to the environment and second in an increased probability of death.

The term senescence is generally used to mean ageing accompanied by a decline in bodily faculties, sensibilities and energies. Dorian Gray aged chronologically but only his portrait disclosed the changes of senescence (Hawker, 1974).

Theories of ageing

Broadly speaking there are two major theories about the mechanisms of ageing: one proposes that ageing, like development and growth, is pre-ordained and genetically controlled through a biological clock; the other suggests that the major factor is not genetic but is due to errors occurring randomly in cells throughout the body. There is, however, no conclusive evidence in support of either theory.

Nor is it known whether the ageing of organs (e.g. skin, teeth and bone) is due to processes occurring independently in the organs themselves, or to blood-borne agents. The immunological theory of ageing postulates that random changes (mutations) occurring in lymphoid cells produce antibodies which then pass via the bloodstream and attack different tissues throughout the body – as an auto-immune process. More research is required to elucidate these fundamental problems of gerontology.

The relation of ageing to disease

Clinicians have long been aware that the age and sex distribution of many diseases are more or less the same from year to year and from country to country. Moreover it is known that many diseases such as diabetes, psoriasis and gout are, in part, genetically determined, and that environmental factors do play a role in the onset, but more particularly in the remission and reassertion of certain diseases. One scientist has in fact argued that several diseases with known genetic- and age-dependency are in fact due to an auto-immune attack as in the immunological theory of ageing.

The future and ageing

Although interest in ageing dates from biblical times, scientific work on gerontology is only just starting. Time and patience will be required to elucidate ageing processes, but a salutary warning may not be misplaced. Although the understanding of the biological processes of ageing and their therapeutic control may lead ultimately to improved vistas of life for the individual, it could add an intolerable burden to a world already troubled by pollution, over-population and the stresses of modern life.

CHANGES ATTRIBUTABLE TO AGEING

The most significant change that occurs as a process of ageing is a reduction in physiological reserves with a potential for a corresponding diminution in recuperative powers in illness or following an accident or other forms of stress.

Physical signs of ageing – greying hair, the changing appearance of the human body, loss of skin elasticity and the formation of wrinkles – all these are visible signs of ageing. However, the person inhabiting this ageing body usually feels exactly the same person that he was when he was young. It is only when he looks in the mirror that he is reminded of his chronological age.

Normal intelligence, sexual capacity, the potential for making relationships with others, do not decline with age in healthy individuals. Physical endurance does decline, but much decrease in fitness and vitality is due to current lifestyles. As we grow older we demand increasingly less of ourselves. There is a progressive reduction in physical activity on the assumption that we become physically less capable. Research has shown that, physiologically, older people's need for exercise is greater than in younger age-groups, and an active mode of life and regular physical activity are essential requirements if physical endurance, health and fitness are to be maintained at their optimum level.

Let us consider some of the changes associated with ageing.

Central nervous system

'The human brain does not shrink, wilt, perish or deteriorate with age. It normally continues to function well through as many as nine decades' (Comfort, 1977).

The brain cells are the longest lived of all the body cells, lasting each person until death. If mental deterioration does occur with time, it is either due to inadequacies in the cerebral vascular circulation or is associated with abnormal areas of neuropathology in the cerebral cortex. Given good health, there is no progressive decline in intelligence in old age. The most characteristic mental changes are associated with memory and learning ability. Memory for recent events is affected by ageing; however, long-term memory still functions well.

Learning when young is rapid and there is usually great capacity for perfect recall, but in older people learning tends to be slower. It has been a traditionally accepted maxim that 'you can't teach an old dog new tricks', but in recent years researchers have been paying more attention to the employment of older people. They have found that although an older worker will take longer to learn a new technique, once learned, the speed achieved is in time comparable with that of a younger person. The younger person, in the absence of previous experience, is able to perform the task spontaneously, whereas an older person with former experience of similar tasks will be inhibited initially by conditioned reflexes and habitual patterns.

It is important to remember that there is no universal blueprint for ageing; mental function and capability will vary from one person to another. Manifestations of mental change may be ascribed less to physiological changes than to poor health and the impoverishment of the individual lifestyles of many elderly people in terms of isolation, boredom, lack of purpose and previous education.

Peripheral nervous system

There is some reduction in the body's perceptual sensitivity in old age and reaction to pain may be altered. There is now evidence to suggest that the pain threshold increases in older people and that sensitivity to pain is reduced, although all through life women have a higher level of pain sensitivity than men.

The special senses

Hearing By the age of 60 most people have lost a great deal of their capacity to detect high-frequency sound, but this is not on the whole a handicap since the sound frequency of ordinary conversational speech is fairly low. Deafness is a common problem for older people and lack of normal two-way communication can produce many problems. Fatalistic acceptance of this is to be avoided – the person with a hearing aid should be encouraged to use it and remedial measures taken if wax is a problem.

Smell and taste There is a close relationship between the senses of smell and taste, and deterioration in one is almost invariably followed by similar deterioration in the other.

A large percentage of older people have a reduced sense of smell, although many retain their appreciation of these senses throughout life.

Eyesight is at its peak in childhood and slowly decreases with age and the lens thereafter gradually loses its elasticity. Around the age of 40 and onward there is a gradual reduction in visual fields, a higher threshold of light stimulation and a slowing of dark adaptation. Spectacles are usually needed for close work. The older person requires greater illumination (frequently up to eight times that required by a younger person) to see adequately and more time than a younger one to adjust when moving from the light into a darker room.

The development of a ring of opacity at the corneal margin called the 'arcus senilis' may occur, but this is of no significant importance and may be absent altogether in many individuals. Loss of orbital fat in older people gives the eyes a sunken appearance.

Speech The ability to communicate remains vital throughout life. In old age the voice becomes restricted in range and power diminishes. Integrated speech patterning may become more difficult – there may be pauses during speech and these pauses may become longer as age increases. Thought processes tend to become externalised and actions may be vocalised (although this is not necessarily a manifestation of old age!).

Cardiovascular system

In old people cardiac output is less during activity than in chronologically younger age-groups and this reduces the level of work-load that can be undertaken. In studies that have been done it has been found that the normal heart of an elderly person is characterised by a gradual decrease in adaptation to effort. Hence the need to maintain physical exercise to improve cardiovascular performance and to reduce the load on the heart.

Decisions regarding the management and control of systemic blood pressure in older people tend to vary. In the past low blood pressure in elderly people was considered, as in younger age-groups, to be a therapeutic necessity but the result of this was that many suffered severe giddiness due to hypotension, becoming as a result severely disabled. If the older person has moderate and widespread arterial changes, hypertension is necessary to maintain blood flow to the central nervous system.

Calcification

Calcium is deposited in new places in the body's tissues while in other areas it is reduced.

Calcification is common in the costal cartilages and by reducing their spring the thoracic cage becomes less elastic. The lift of the ribs in inspiration and recoil during expiration is reduced and ventilatory capacity is diminished.

Calcification of the thyroid cartilage produces an alteration in the voice and there is a tendency too for the cartilage to fracture easily and this fact must be remembered when handling the neck.

Calcium may also be laid down in the trachea and bronchi, in the aorta and the peripheral vessels.

At the same time there may be a loss of calcium from the bones which then become porous and brittle and may fracture after fairly trivial trauma. This condition of the bones is called osteoporosis and is common in women after the menopause as endocrines play a part in the process, as does prolonged inactivity such as complete bedrest.

Musculoskeletal system

Articular cartilage becomes yellowish in colour with age and its elasticity and compressibility lessens. The discs between the vertebrae become thinner and there is usually a slight loss of height, which amounts to about 12.5mm (½in) every 20 years after the age of 40.

Joints may show many histological changes with age, but very old people frequently have very good joint function.

The musculature of older people shows progressive weakness and less bulk as the muscles begin to lose fibres and by the time a person is old the loss of muscle tissue is usually noticeable. It is believed that up to the age of 30 the number of muscle fibres remains the same as at birth. However, active, well-nourished elderly people preserve their strength to a remarkable degree. Suitable exercise still leads to an increase in the size of muscle fibres, which tends to offset the loss in numbers.

DEMOGRAPHICAL CHANGES IN THE POPULATION

A century ago a boy at birth could expect to live to 41 and a girl to 45. Today a boy can expect to live to 69 and a girl to 75. This transformation in life expectancy is affecting the population structure not only in Britain but in *all* the developed countries in the world.

In our own country we have a situation never before encountered in our history. Not only is the pensionable population growing three times faster than the rest of the population as a whole, but at the same time there has been a dramatic increase in those in their eighth, ninth and even tenth decade, and this trend is likely to continue.

In 1901 1 person in every 20 was over 65; by 1981 this number had increased to approximately 1 in 7. For those over the age of 75, the respective figures are 1 in every 82 at the turn of the century and 1 in every 18 today. By the end of the century people over 85 years of age are expected to number 845 000, an increase of roughly 300 000 on today's figure.

Because women live longer than men there are twice as many women as men over the age of 75. Many of these are single, reflecting the high casualty figures of men killed in World War I.

Dependency ratio

The high birth ratio at the beginning of the century has been followed by a very much lower one and as a result there are relatively fewer people to support the dependent age-groups, which are the very young and the very old.

Life expectancy

It should be made clear that people are not living to be older, but it does mean that old age has become possible for a much larger number.

Life expectancy for people over the age of 65 has increased but little in the last 80 years (in 1911 a man aged 65 could expect to live a further 11 years compared with 12 now; a woman aged 65 could expect to live 12 more years as against 16 years now).

Medicated survival

This revolutionary increase in the number of old people has been brought about as a result of the successful fight against illness and disease in the young caused by vast improvements in social conditions (sanitation, nutrition, housing and working conditions), as well as the great reduction in infant mortality due to improvements in neonatal and obstetric care. Comfort (1977) says, 'Medicine has done nothing whatever to alter the human life span, but it has been strikingly successful in making us live to the end of it.'

Morbidity

The major health problems of the late twentieth century are very different from those at the beginning of the century. With the control or disappearance of the lethal diseases of childhood – tuberculosis and infections – it is the degenerative long-term conditions, such as cardiovascular, cerebrovascular, renal or respiratory insufficiency, neurological disorders and diseases of the musculoskeletal system, which contribute to disability in older age. Because of their longer life-span women are particularly vulnerable, living on with increasing frailty and accumulated pathology.

Such conditions have one important characteristic in common in the fact that many of their sequelae have to be lived with because the underlying cause cannot be cured. However, a considerable number are amenable to treatment and management if detected early enough. Unfortunately, a high proportion of unknown disability exists among elderly people and it is known that a large number make few demands on their doctors unless they are really ill or have begun to be so disabled that mobility and independence are seriously threatened.

REFERENCES

Comfort, A. (1977). *A Good Age.* Mitchell Beazley, London.
Gore, I. (1979). *Age and Vitality.* Unwin Paperbacks, London.
Hawker, M. (1974). *Geriatrics for Physiotherapists and the Allied Professions,* p. 17. Faber and Faber, London.

Chapter Two

SOME ASPECTS OF AGEING

Ageing is a continuing life process which involves change. The majority of older people are able to cope with this process and with the adjustments to such demands as an abrupt ending of active employment and a severely reduced income, or bereavement and widowhood. Much help comes from friends and neighbours and from families who continue to provide the supreme comfort and support.

HEALTH

'The ability to accept and adapt to the altered conditions of later life, depend in great measure on retention of health and vigour. Health in old age starts with middle age' (*Health for Old Age*, 1970).

It could be suggested that attitudes to health should start even earlier, for if leisure in retirement is to be enjoyed it is important to maintain fitness in earlier years. Within reason minds and bodies respond better to being overstretched rather than under-used and as Irene Gore (1979) has pointed out, 'most of us live our lives out of condition – not ill, but not really well'.

Regular exercise has a benefical effect on both mind and body and much research has been undertaken on the effects of exercise in increasing general physical fitness, mobility and stamina and on improving mental states and feelings of well-being. It has been shown that a substantial improvement in physical function, equal to 20 biological years, can be achieved by graded training over 6 to 10 weeks in 70-year-old males (Thompson, 1979). Mental disability is far more likely to arise from lack of stimulus and interest, and withdrawal from life, than from the effects of organic disease.

Self-knowledge, personal responsibility and control of such social habits as smoking, over-indulgence in alcohol, over-eating and obesity, are crucial factors in maintaining health in later years. The importance of pre-retirement training and education in earlier years on the use of leisure, so that interests and skills can be developed and boredom and mental stagnation avoided, is only beginning to be recognised. 'Decent nutrition, regular and sufficient physical activity and mental stimulation, involvement in life, contact with the world and due attention paid to any untoward symptoms – these are the basic requirements for young and old alike' (Gore, 1979).

RELATIONSHIPS

It is important that we, as a society, recognise our interdependence upon one another and learn to cultivate genuine relationships with other people, not only for the stimulus and pleasure that this can bring but also so that we can establish a network of support and concern in time of need. Nor should these relationships be limited to one's own age-group. It is important, if attitudes and ideas are to remain flexible, that the generation gaps be well bridged so that people have the opportunity to learn from each other and recognise individual needs.

Employment can mask isolation and it is essential to develop relationships well before retirement age. The death of a marriage partner in whom all one's emotional dependence has been centred can have disastrous effects without the help of friends to provide support during the bereavement stage.

Longer survival means that husbands and wives live longer together. Most couples arrive at retirement age totally unprepared for this long period of close domestic proximity after years when the pattern of domestic life has been dictated by the demands of the breadwinner's regular job. Even for couples who eventually reach dual fulfilment in retirement, adjustments need to be made. Where there is lack of self-awareness by one or both partners, or incompatibility in the relationship, then the problems of living together over the years, perhaps with the added difficulties of diminishing capability, are indeed formidable. The problems will be further exacerbated if the couple are without friends or neighbours to give help.

Personal relationships

Being physically and emotionally close, showing tenderness and enjoying sexual activity, are all elements of a loving relationship and are essential human needs at any age of life. Even if sexual activity is impaired by ill-health or disability, it is a mistake to believe it to be the end of sensuality and of being valued as a person.

Unfortunately, as Alex Comfort (1977) has said, it has long been an accepted social image that the old 'are and should be asexual'. However, biology has not established a mandatory age for sexual retirement and studies of people of 65 and over have shown that sexual activity continues and can, in fact, be life long, although for some libido and performance do diminish.

This taboo subject has until recently been riddled with misconceptions but now in our more permissive society there is every expectation that attitudes will change and that rising generations of older people will be less influenced by folklore than in the past.

It is essential that professional carers show understanding and sensitivity, so that the normal human needs of older people living in hospital or residential care should not be diminished or denied. The importance of privacy and the right to continue or develop relationships should be recognised and accommodated whenever possible.

BEREAVEMENT

Few people are fully prepared for this experience, for as it has been said, 'bereavement brings about a crisis of loss, probably the most severe crisis in human existence' (Parkes, 1975). The loss of a partner in any committed relationship in which life has been shared, means the collapse of mutual support and the complete disruption of an established way of life. For those who are elderly the association with the dead person has usually been lengthy and it is indeed hard to build up life again and establish new relationships. Nor have the majority of older people, in comparison with younger age-groups, such outlets as a job or career to help alleviate grief.

Women live longer than men and have therefore an approximate 70 per cent expectation of widowhood, but in spite of this it is rare in our society that there will have been any preparation for this likely outcome and many wives are left unable to cope with so many practical details which throughout their married lives have remained the husband's particular responsibility.

Until fairly recently there have been few studies by psychiatrists on reactions to bereavement. Grief, which is the normal reaction to loss, can be regarded as 'a distinct psychological process, characterised by a number of stages which blend into and replace each other' (Parkes, 1975). It is only after the last of these stages has been reached that recovery can take place. Although most people come through this experience without need for professional help, for some individuals bereavement remains unresolved and as a result it can have a detrimental effect on physical and mental health.

Bereavement is a process which cannot be hurried. Time is the crucial factor. It is essential, in order that the bereaved person can realise loss, for feelings to emerge into consciousness.

Expressing grief is not always easy. In the past, ritual observations of mourning had great psychological value, but in Western society, unfortunately, such customs are increasingly on the decline. A general atmosphere of acceptance of the need to mourn by family, friends and neighbours, is crucial if the process is to be completed and the bereaved person enabled to return to life again. However, many people find it difficult to accept this need to mourn because of their feelings of embarrassment in the presence of the newly bereaved. Yet not only does the inability to accept grief and mourning leave people unprepared for eventual loss themselves, but it also means that they will lack the necessary maturity to help others.

Suppression of grief can mean an interruption to the normal stages of bereavement and the person concerned may complain of ill-health or suffer from general emotional disturbances, or even withdrawal into a life of isolation and apathy.

One of the most important functions of supporting friends and family is for someone closely concerned to provide reassurance, after an appropriate period of time, that grieving may cease and thus the bereaved person is set free to rebuild life once more. Parkes (1975) says, 'To some extent, grieving is seen as a duty to the dead and it may take an outsider to point out that the duty is now done.'

LONELINESS

Although over two million of the retired live alone this does not mean that all suffer from loneliness. Many are independent out-going citizens who live alone from choice. Nor is loneliness a situation that occurs only in later life – a person may be lonely at any age. As people grow into extreme old age, however, they tend to outlive their relatives, friends and contemporaries and some may suffer from loneliness and social isolation.

Bereavement, as discussed already, is probably the most isolating experience. Increasing infirmity which saps energy reserves, loss of mobility, problems of hearing or vision, inadequate housing, distance from shops and lack of transport, and diminished income are other factors which make it increasingly difficult to maintain contacts and friendships.

A regular job, so often an antidote to loneliness in earlier life, is seldom available for retired people. For this reason work or day centres, pop-in parlours, lunch and other clubs, mobile shops and libraries for the housebound, are some of the facilities needed if loneliness is to be combated.

Some people throughout life have found social relationships difficult and such a person in old age may tend to become increasingly eccentric in habits, possibly withdrawing from social life and living as a recluse. Offers of help are frequently refused and as a result both mental and physical health deteriorate and the old person can suffer from neglect, apathy and malnutrition.

DEATH AND TERMINAL ILLNESS

In the past, mortality rates of children and adolescents were high and as a result death was a familiar experience to most families and accepted with resignation. Today we have a very different situation. There are now no significant causes of death before middle age. Even those causes of death which do occur in youth, do so infrequently. Mortality now rarely occurs before the age of 45 and the incidence of death is largely concentrated in old age. Thus death and dying are no longer familiar experiences for younger age-groups and to society as a whole death has become a taboo subject, something to be feared and staved off at all cost, rather than the natural and appropriate culmination of a full life.

However, as Alex Comfort (1977) says, 'later life is not often preoccupied with death . . . and all that the proximity of death does to age is to add value to living'.

Rather it is the process of living which causes anxiety. Most people would prefer a quick death rather than having to undergo a period of prolonged illness, which many fear might be accompanied by such problems as pain, incontinence or mental confusion. For the older person there is the additional anxiety of being a burden to those around.

Traditionally the process of dying has been regarded as part of death rather than part of life. Many in the medical profession, orientated towards the diagnosis, cure or alleviation of diseases, feel that they have an extremely limited role to play in this process. In the study *Life before Death* based on a survey of people in the last year of their lives, the authors found that of the total number of this sample, only 2 per cent had died in teaching hospitals, suggesting that doctors are rarely confronted by death in their training and as a result may feel helpless in this situation, thinking there is little or nothing they can do (Cartwright, 1973).

When someone is in the terminal stage of illness, comfort and peace of mind are all important and all concerned will need an understanding and sensitive approach. Skilled medical and other professional support are essential so that an appropriate plan of management can be developed to meet each patient's individual needs.

Problems of intractable incontinence can be controlled by good management; pain when present can be alleviated; and confusion, so often the way of retreat from an untenable situation rather than an organic condition, is frequently reversible if the patient's individual needs are recognised and he is made to feel included and involved in the life around him.

The growth in recent years of special centres for the management of terminal care has shown the way in which a 'good death' can be achieved, either at home or in hospital. The control of symptoms in terminal cancer to alleviate pain and suffering is now recognised as a speciality in its own right and is increasingly becoming a part of medical teaching. Much of the work that has been carried out in this field is equally appropriate to the relief of distress in other terminal situations.

It is crucial that all those concerned with the care and support of the terminally ill should work together, and this includes the patient, family and friends, as well as professional carers. The person who is dying frequently feels isolated, surrounded by a conspiracy of silence, both sides protecting each other from the truth uppermost in their thoughts. It may be easier, at least initially, for the patient to share anxieties with another member of the team with whom he has established a personal rapport.

Professional carers too, need the mutual support of each other in what can often be extremely stressful situations. Moreover, as Cicely Saunders (1978) says, 'with advances in technical medicine there is much anxiety that staff may be involved in treatments which they feel may only prolong the patient's distress'.

This is a dilemma which has relevance for the physiotherapist, whose services are so often called upon when pneumonia is diagnosed. Each situation must be judged individually and it is in this sort of circumstance that multidisciplinary discussion is so vital, so that the implications of a particular therapeutic policy can be talked over and an appropriate plan evolved for each patient.

Working together in this way in cases of terminal illness, all involved can derive not only fuller understanding of the needs of the dying person, but greater insight into their own strengths and weaknesses and personal philosophy.

PUTTING THINGS IN PERSPECTIVE

1. Old age is not a disease

Growing old is a normal process in which we are all involved. *Being* old can have its difficulties, one of which is illness, but old age and illness are not synonymous. In most Western countries old age is associated with illness and the person who is old is thought to be sick. This is because the sick old are particularly noticeable while the active elderly are often not thought of as being aged since 'those who manage well live their lives unremarked' (*Arrangement for Old Age*, 1969).

For care-giving personnel, particularly those working in hospitals or residential homes and involved with the day-to-day problems of severely disabled elderly people, it is important to remember, if perspective is to be maintained, that at any one time only 6 per cent of the elderly are in any form of institution. Some 94 per cent are living in the community and although approximately 13 per cent of these may be housebound, the remainder are managing to live more or less active and independent lives. The point has been well illustrated in an article by Professor Bernard Isaacs (1974) in which he says, 'I discovered to my astonishment that 80 per cent of old people did not suffer from physical impairment, while 90 per cent were free of mental decrepitude. Continuing my exploration I found that the number of old people who were not incontinent, who had never had a stroke, a fall or a pressure sore, who were not housebound, chair-bound or bedbound, ran into millions.'

2. Attitudes and assumptions

Society's preoccupation with calendar age does its older citizens a grave disservice. The habit of judging individual potential by age rather than by personal capability is a manifestation of discrimination and prejudice that when applied to older people is known as *ageism*.

Ageism reflects society's negative and patronising attitude towards its older members who have come to be regarded as a race apart, no longer participants in the mainstream of life nor subject to the same thoughts and feelings as the rest of society.

There are several reasons for this attitude. One stems from the universal fear of ageing and the attempts we make to avoid the reality that all of us must grow older and eventually die.

Another factor is the emphasis placed in our modern industrial economy on productive capacity and technological expertise. It is indeed paradoxical that by the introduction of compulsory retirement at a mandatory age, society not only deprives older people of occupational status by 'ejecting them from a citizenship based on work' (Comfort, 1977) regardless of individual competence and experience, but at the same time by definition they become an old person. And this transformation is not based on biological or physical change but on a political and economic transformation laid upon people arbitrarily after a fixed number of years.

It is not the person who changes on his 65th birthday but society's attitude to him and this may well affect the individual's view of himself so that in time he may come to regard himself as old, spent and useless, lacking the potential for continued human growth and development. For the growing number of elderly members of ethnic minorities in this country, how much greater the stress suffered by those discriminated against not only by age but also by the colour of their skins?

OLDER PEOPLE ARE PEOPLE

We must recognise the process of ageing not as a static concept but as a continuum of growth and development, 'a process of addition rather than subtraction, of a growing maturity rather than loss of youth, of evolution rather than dissolution. If such a concept removes the pernicious, if subconscious, obsession with calendar age . . . the more readily we shall go on participating in life' (Gore, 1979). The effects of ageing vary so much from individual to individual that functional rather than chronological age is a more realistic criterion.

As discussed in Chapter 1, the older person feels very little different from when he was young. Although external appearances change with age, memory, sexuality, activity, capacity for relationships and zest for living will normally be life long in healthy individuals. Elderly people do not all want the same things but they do need the freedom to choose their own lifestyle, to have reasonable health, companionship, purpose for living and be able to influence events. These needs are no different from any other member of society.

IMPLICATIONS FOR THE FUTURE

If retirement years are to provide opportunities for individual growth and fulfilment, then it is imperative that society takes a long hard look at the largely stereotyped and passive role it has given older people and it is equally important that older people themselves refuse to take on the part assigned to them by society 'who wish them puppet-like to play the scene their way' (Warnock, 1983).

Within our midst we have a priceless resource of experience, talents, wisdom and knowledge, most of which is wastefully squandered by denying retired people opportunities to contribute to their society.

The increasing emphasis on community care, together with the growing pressures on statutory resources, must result in closer co-ordination of professional, voluntary and informal effort if breakdown of independence of vulnerable people of all age-groups is to be prevented. It would appear logical that by harnessing the experience and energies of recently retired people and by sharing with them professional expertise, the caring agencies could be provided with a network of ground support which would enable them to make the most of service development. Many retired people are already involved in voluntary organisations and community support groups, such as tenants' associations or good neighbour schemes. It is a known fact that the vast majority of care and support given to frail elderly people is provided on an informal basis by friends and neighbours. All that is required to extend the principle and for society to use the untapped human resources within its midst is a fundamental change in current attitudes and assumptions.

But if retired people are to live purposeful lives, not only opportunities, but resources and support are essential to make it so. In this materialistic, youth-orientated society of ours, with its emphasis on economic survival, what range of options are available to give life satisfaction and to meet individual needs, including the special needs of those with different cultural and religious backgrounds?

REFERENCES

Arrangement for Old Age (1969). Consumers' Association, London.
Cartwright, A. (1973). *Life Before Death.* Routledge and Kegan Paul, London.
Comfort, A. (1977). *A Good Life.* Mitchell Beazley, London.
Gore, I. (1979). *Age and Vitality.* Unwin Paperbacks, London.
Health for Old Age (1970). Consumers' Association, London.
Isaacs, B. (1974). Standing old people on their heads. *Community Health*, **6**.
Parkes, C. M. (1975). *Bereavement.* Penguin Books, Harmondsworth.
Saunders, C. (1978). Care of the Dying. In *An Ageing Population* (ed Carver, V. and Liddiard, P.). Hodder and Stoughton, London.
Thompson, K. M. (1979). Even at 65, the 'old' have a capacity for growth. *Modern Geriatrics*, **11**, 49.
Warnock, M . (1983). *The Nature of Choice.* Occasional Paper 8. Age Concern England.

Chapter Three

RETIREMENT IN THE 1980s

With as many as 30 years at their disposal, such factors as employment opportunities, housing, finance, transport, educational and recreational facilities and a host of others will have a direct bearing on the lifestyles of retired people.

EMPLOYMENT OPPORTUNITIES

The current policy of compulsory retirement at a mandatory age, regardless of individual employees' wishes has already been referred to in Chapter 2.

Opportunities for people over retirement age to continue full- or part-time work are extremely limited in the present economic climate. In a time of high unemployment, elderly and handicapped workers are among those who suffer most. In 1921 nearly 80 per cent of men over the age of 65 were still working. In 1971 the numbers had fallen to 16 per cent. Today men over 55 are approximately twice as likely as younger age-groups to become unemployed and the trend is towards shifting the burden of unemployment on to older workers through redundancy and early retirement.

The abolishment of compulsory retirement and the institution of a flexible policy over a range of 10 years from 60 to 70, for example, has been advocated as one answer to age discrimination in employment. Re-deployment, including retraining courses, job sharing, the use of 'flexitime' and sabbaticals, part work and part pension schemes, are other options proposed. Economic changes are forcing a re-examination of currently held attitudes to work and the role it has played in our lives. Given the likely continuation of the current economic situation, there is an urgent need to create acceptable social alternatives for people out of work. Retirement too would become a liberating and attractive option for many employees if pensions could be increased.

Self-help groups of retired and unemployed people with particular skills can provide a valuable resource. For example those with teaching qualifications could help with the educational needs of children and adults in such situations as community colleges or pre-retirement courses. Building workers, another example, could provide a valuable service in home repairs and maintenance for vulnerable people in the community. Services organised under local authorities such as the meals-on-wheels service, good neighbour schemes or organisers of volunteers require personnel and this can be a means of earning a small income. Voluntary agencies frequently need help in developing local community care and support groups, such as care-attendant schemes or day centres.

HOUSING

There can be little doubt that properly designed housing is the most important single factor in the preservation of independence in older people. It can make all the difference between continuing ability to live in the community or the need for residential support in an old people's home, or even hospital.

A high proportion of older people are owner-occupiers although many may live in sub-standard housing and lack such basic amenities as indoor lavatories, hot water or a bathroom.

In recent years there has been an increasing tendency for retired people to move from the towns to what they see as more congenial and attractive environs. In some of the popular retirement areas in coastal resorts at least one-third of the population are elderly and this figure is mounting. Moving house is something that needs to be thought about extremely carefully and if possible plans should be made long before retirement day. Many people are lured away from their familiar neighbourhoods and friendships built up over the years by recollections of an idyllic summer holiday spent in some rural and remote part of the countryside. Once moved to the new locality, such factors as the lack of shops within walking distance, inadequate public transport or a neighbour within hailing distance may pose increasing problems as the years go by.

Independent housing

Although rate rebates and rent allowances help to ensure that retired people are able to meet the basic cost of housing, meeting major capital expenses can prove a continuous worry for many house owners. As families grow up and leave home, some older people find themselves overhoused and they are left with the expense of heating, maintaining and cleaning a house too large for them. Some may find that they have to cope with disability and in such a situation awkward and steep staircases, and no ground floor lavatory, for example, can be particularly handicapping.

Under certain conditions, grants from the local council can be obtained for repairs or improvements to property and even for converting an over-large house into two or more individual dwellings. Adaptations to the home, such as installing a ground floor lavatory or shower, or a stair lift so that disabled people are enabled to continue to live independently in their own homes, are financed through social services departments.

Alternative accommodation

An alternative to continuing to live in one's original if unsuitable home, is to move into some kind of purpose-designed housing for handicapped people, such as 'mobility-housing' – that is, housing suitable for people who have mobility handicaps. Dwellings are frequently grouped together and can include small houses, bungalows or flatlets. Some have the services of a warden, in which case the accommodation is usually referred to as sheltered housing.

Voluntary housing associations, local authorities and, nowadays, the private sector, provide this type of housing and waiting lists can be lengthy since there is a growing demand for such accommodation. Residents must generally be able to look after themselves, although the usual domiciliary support services can be provided where there is a need. Housing authorities are normally separate from health and social service authorities, and the provision of specialised housing is increasingly being recognised as a vital element in the support of older people. It is essential that it is provided within a framework of local community health and social services so that tenants can have the support of all the resources provided by these statutory authorities such as home helps or nursing assistance, if required.

Sheltered housing is either purpose built or older property that has been converted. It consists of self-contained easily maintained living units, each with its own front door. There is often a common room and a visitors' room for overnight use if residents want a relative or friend to stay. Frequently laundry facilities are provided and there is usually some form of emergency call system. There is generally a warden to keep an eye on tenants and provide help in an emergency. Stockport local authority has developed mobile wardens and a radio alarm system (Shegog, 1981).

In many situations sheltered housing facilities are being used primarily to meet inadequate housing needs of elderly people who do not require a daily check on their well-being by the warden and resent 'these inroads into personal privacy' (Eley et al, 1983). Purpose-built sheltered housing is often located away from the centre of the town or village, since building land is more available there. As a result, tenants can be cut off from shops and other amenities and isolated from their local community.

There is a great need to re-examine the role of sheltered housing with its expensive built-in facilities and resident warden service which can help to undermine tenants' confidence and self-reliance.

For the majority of vulnerable people of any age purposefully designed accommodation with background central heating and a telephone are the basic requirements needed. The availability of a caretaker or good neighbour scheme, and the provision of domiciliary services both statutory and voluntary for those requiring help with physical needs, would frequently be a more appropriate answer.

FINANCE

The onset of retirement marks a severe drop in income for the majority of the population. Even those who have been able to cushion themselves against the risk of retirement by means of savings, investments and the provision of an occupational as well as the state retirement pension, have found that their incomes have been severely reduced in recent years because of the effects of inflation. For those who have little but the state retirement pension to rely on, the consequences of inflation have been felt even more keenly and these pensioners are the poorest section of our society.

Retirement pensions

In 1978 the government's new earnings related pension scheme was introduced and it will eventually, after coming to full maturity in 20 years' time, provide improved conditions for many pensioners. However, the scheme will not solve the problem of people already retired or help those due to retire before the end of the century. The retirement pension is paid to women at the age of 60 and men at 65, providing they have retired from full-time work and have paid sufficient national insurance contributions (*Your Rights*, 1983).

Going on working

The retirement pension can be deferred if a person has the opportunity to continue in full-time employment. At the age of 70 for a man (65 for a woman) the pension can then be drawn and there will be no restrictions on the length of time the pensioner continues working or on the amount earned. However, the majority of the population does not have the opportunity to continue in their present employment after retirement age and alternative full-time work is difficult to obtain. If part-time work is taken on in order to supplement the state retirement pension, then this pension will be reduced if the pensioner earns more than a certain amount a week. This earning restriction applies for the first five years of retirement and is called the 'earnings rule'.

The application of the 'earnings rule' not only acts as a disincentive to older people to continue working, but is further evidence of age discrimination referred to in Chapter 2.

Supplementary benefits

The DHSS supplementary pension is a means-tested benefit designed to bring the recipient's income up to a certain level ('the minimum standard of living that the Government consider necessary at a particular time'). Special levels apply for people living with their family, or if they are in hospital or residential home. In addition, extra allowances can be obtained to help with rates, rents or mortgage interest. Rents and general rates are no longer covered by supplementary benefit. Instead, help comes from the local authority under the housing benefit scheme.

A pensioner on supplementary benefit can receive allowances to help with heating costs, laundry expenses in case of illness or incontinence, and for special diets.

Practically two-and-a-half million people over retirement age are in receipt of supplementary pensions and, therefore, by definition are close to the poverty line; another 600 000 are thought to be eligible for such help, but are not claiming it. This is partly because some may be ignorant of what is available or, and this is particularly significant, because they are reluctant to accept what they feel to be charity. Living on incomes on and around the supplementary benefit level allows little room for manoeuvre and imposes on large numbers of elderly people severe constraints on individual quality of life.

Many members of ethnic minorities, who will fail to make the full national insurance contributions before retirement and will therefore have to depend very largely on supplementary benefit, fail to claim it because they are totally unaware of their entitlement.

Non-contributory benefits

Attendance allowance

This allowance represents the main form of financial assistance additional to the retirement pension available to elderly people whose mental or physical disability is of six months' duration or over and who need frequent personal attention. The allowance is paid at two rates:

Invalid care allowance This benefit is paid to anyone of working age (other than a married woman living with or supported by her husband) who gives up work to look after a person in receipt of the attendance allowance. It is, therefore, of limited value to those over retirement age, but can be of assistance to a daughter or daughter-in-law providing help to an elderly parent, as long as the daughter or daughter-in-law in question is single, widowed or divorced.

Mobility allowance This benefit is paid to disabled people who are unable, or virtually unable, to walk. It cannot be claimed over the age of 65, although those already in receipt of the allowance before their 65th birthday will continue to be eligible until the age of 75. Not only does this inequitable regulation preclude from benefit large numbers of disabled people over the age of 75 (when mobility problems become most acute), and bars from eligibility people whose disability does not manifest itself until after the age of 65, but it also causes others to 'have to make a painful adjustment to the loss at 75 of a significant part of their income' (Topliss, 1982).

MOBILITY

Without the ability and resources to be mobile, elderly people, as with any other members of the population, are cut off from normal social life, from going to the shops, for example, from visiting friends or getting to the library or local pub or church. Since 86.5 per cent of people over 65 do not hold a driving licence and 76 per cent are not living in a car-owning household, they are far more dependent on walking and on public transport than the rest of the community. For those who are disabled or extremely old and frail, special facilities are required if they are to be enabled to live a fulfilling social ife and to reach the services they need.

Environment

The availability and accessibility of local facilities are of increasing importance as one gets older. High kerbs, unramped pavements, steps too steep, long underpasses, insufficient crossing time at pedestrian crossings and the ever-growing volume of traffic all act as barriers to mobility. The development of shopping precincts has many advantages, but getting to and from the town centre is not always easy and the local corner shop is a facility that is fast disappearing.

Access to public buildings

Section 4 of the Chronically Sick and Disabled Persons Act 1970 makes provision for the needs of disabled people visiting buildings open to the general public. Such things as ramps, the use of car parking and lavatory facilities, must be included whenever practicable and reasonable in all new buildings and premises.

Unfortunately, not all authorities and private development are as yet prepared to follow this policy. The announcement in October 1983 by the Minister for the Disabled of the establishment of the Access Committee for England to study the issues involved is encouraging.

Public transport

'The trends in passenger transport in this country, as in many other industrialised countries, are dominated by the growth in private motoring' (Norman, 1977). As a result services grow more infrequent, unreliable and expensive and in many rural areas there may be no service at all. The practical difficulties for older people of using buses include the distance to and from bus stops, long waiting periods, and the physical problems involved in getting on and off a vehicle and maintaining balance as it accelerates. Dial-a-bus and local taxi schemes using converted mini-buses, station-wagon type cars and ambulances, post-buses which carry both mail and passengers, and the use of volunteer drivers on scheduled public services are some examples where local initiative in co-operation with the appropriate authorities have produced some alternative solutions. But much more is needed.

British Rail has done a good deal to meet the needs of severely disabled travellers, but little for those who are mobile but elderly and frail. The absence of porters, the inadequate number of luggage trolleys and the almost complete disappearance of platform benches add to the difficulties of train travel, particularly when luggage has to be carried.

Travel concessions

British Rail offers a 'senior citizen railcard' at a reasonable cost to people of pensionable age and this enables older people to buy tickets over the following 12 months at half the usual price.

Many local authorities provide cheaper or free bus fares for pensioners, but the conditions vary from one locality to another and in some parts of the country no concessions at all are provided. This is particularly the case in rural areas where generally the journeys are longest and buses scarcer. Ever-increasing bus fares are causing particular hardship to retired people on a fixed pension in areas where no travel concessions have been granted and there is a great need to rationalise the present system of concessionary fares.

Access to domiciliary and hospital services

Distances from family doctors' practices have increased with the centralisation of premises and this has created problems for older people who have to rely on public transport to get to and from their general practitioner.

The demands on hospital ambulance services are well known. A high percentage of attendances are for out-patient physiotherapy and well over half the people involved are over 65. Day hospitals put extra pressures on ambulance services and because of the difficulties of bringing patients on time, day hospitals can be under-deployed with consequent implications for professional staff concerned. Much time is spent by patients travelling to the day hospital or physiotherapy department with resulting disruption to their daily life.

There is a great need for a systematic reappraisal of ambulance transport to identify requirements of individual services. The often duplicating demands on transport and personnel by a day hospital and physiotherapy department need to be examined and, where possible, alternative and more appropriate solutions, such as the development of a community physiotherapy service, found.

Demands on social services departments' transport resources are numerous and include not only taking elderly people to day centres and to residential homes for day care, but also transporting schoolchildren, mentally and physically handicapped adults to special centres, providing clients with meals-on-wheels and collecting and distributing aids and appliances for disabled people. Many of the demands on transport and the problems of organisation of resources are familiar to those of the ambulance service.

EDUCATION

The development of a satisfying lifestyle early in life will do a great deal to ensure that life in retirement will be purposeful and fulfilling. For some who have had an absorbing interest outside their work, retirement cannot come quickly enough to give them the time to pursue and develop their particular interest. For others, and this applies especially to men, the sudden cessation of the work-ordered day leaves a void which can be difficult or impossible to fill. Education to date does little to prepare people for living, by developing individual interests and potential, so latent talents and skills remain hidden and unrecognised and for many the long 'bonus' years of retirement can be just a matter of filling in time.

Adult education can be of particular value to older people for it can provide opportunity for the development of a wide range of intellectual, practical and creative skills and at the same time it is a means of bringing people together so that fresh social contacts can be made and friendships developed. Educational provision for older people in this country has some way yet to go. In the USA educational courses for older age-groups have been developed in a number of colleges and universities and in France a focal point for continuing education of elderly people is through the University of the Third Age founded in 1972. In Britain local Third Age University groups are beginning to be organised in various parts of the country. In the United Kingdom local education authorities provide evening and some day classes for adults of all ages and a variety of courses are planned.

Usually, reduced fees are offered for people of retirement age and sometimes transport can be arranged. Health education and keep-fit classes are other facilities specially planned for retired people. Other educational bodies involved are the extra-mural studies departments of many universities. The Open University has particular advantages for elderly people since a large part of the students' work can be done at home. A significant number of retired people, deprived of educational opportunities earlier in life, have been enabled to continue their education and to achieve degree status.

Pre-retirement education

Retirement marks an important transition stage in many people's lives. The loss of a daily ordered routine, the rewarding contact with colleagues and fellow workers, and a considerable drop in income – all these and many other factors need careful thought and discussion if retirement is not to mean boredom, loneliness and lack of purpose. At present only 6 per cent of employees approaching retirement receive any preparation. Many of these courses are organised by employers in collaboration with adult education agencies and voluntary bodies. The Pre-Retirement Association has been active in this field since 1964.

Special attention needs to be given to preparing members of ethnic groups for retirement in this country since the problems for them are very different from those of the indigenous population.

HOLIDAYS

For many of today's retired, born at the beginning of the century, holidays were a luxury they could ill afford. For the rising generation of older people a holiday is looked upon as an accepted way of life and even in spite of reduced circumstances it is usually possible to find some means of getting away on holiday even though both the time of year and the actual location may not be the primary choice. Holiday options are extremely varied. For those who are active there are, for example, walking tours of graded ability. Educational holidays ranging from a weekend or longer are run on a variety of topics. These are frequently organised by colleges of adult education and this includes the Open University where a one-week residential summer school is held for all first-year students.

Group holiday schemes are arranged by clubs for their elderly members, such as the OAP Association. Holidays abroad are a possibility and many travel firms are offering three-month holidays abroad very reasonably. Many of these are off-season, which means that the weather can be unreliable. Holidays for elderly and disabled people may be provided or subsidised by the local authority and help may also be obtained with travelling. Many voluntary bodies acting as agents for the local authority undertake the organisation of these holidays.

Travel concessions, particularly travel by rail, can be used with great advantage and the holder of a senior citizen railcard is able to obtain reduced fares for travel to, and in, certain European countries, in addition to the UK.

AGE IS OPPORTUNITY

Retirement and the leisure it brings can offer opportunities which have never been possible during a lifetime of full employment. As mentioned already, if we are to remain a viable society, it is essential that we use the experience and skills of our older members in valid and worthwhile ways.

It is also essential that retired people themselves take individual responsibility to develop latent potential talents, extend interests and involvement and ensure as far as possible personal health and well-being. Equally important is the need for retired people to join with others both at neighbourly or more formal local and national levels in order to provide mutual support for each other in time of difficulty, to highlight specific needs or gaps in services, and finally, as members of the voting population, to influence social policies on which their own and coming generations of older people's fulfilment depends.

REFERENCES

Eley, R. et al (1983). Square pegs, round holes? *Health Trends*, **15**, 68.

Norman, A. (1977). *Transport and the Elderly*. National Corporation for the Care of Old People, London.

Shegog, R.F.A. (ed.) (1981). *The Impending Crisis of Old Age*. Nuffield Provincial Hospitals Trust, Oxford University Press, Oxford.

Topliss, E. (1982). *Social Responses to Handicap*. Longman Group Limited, London.

Your Rights (1983). Age Concern England.

Chapter Four

WHEN HELP IS NEEDED

As already discussed, the considerable number of people who, for purely actuarial reasons, are regarded as of 'pensionable age' are not socially or biologically old. It is those of 75 years of age and upwards, rather than the much larger group of people between 65 and 74, who are most likely to need help.

'We cannot take the pain out of the fact that human beings are not immortal or indefinitely disease-proof or that illness accumulates as we age' (Comfort, 1977). Nor can each individual avoid the fact that throughout his lifetime, he will be subject to periods of change and transition, demanding in greater or lesser degree personal and social readjustments. It is important to remember that the differences between individual elderly people are far greater than those which supposedly distinguish them from the rest of the population.

How people respond to seemingly impossible odds depends upon an individual's inner resources, personal resilience and expectations. Some will continue to manage, others will succumb to far less pressure.

Most old people, even when handicapped to some degree, manage to look after themselves in their own homes with the help of spouses, relatives and neighbours. Frail equilibrium can be undermined by a variety of precipitating factors such as an acute medical episode, increasing disability or a life crisis such as the death of a spouse. In such situations help, both immediate and long-term, in the form of treatment and management will be required and, if necessary, 24-hour support and practical assistance. To avoid the disruptive effects on elderly people of displacement from a familiar environment, the help provided will need, ideally, to be home-based so that family ties and neighbourly links can be maintained.

Such a concept requires a framework of comprehensive domiciliary support covering unsocial hours and weekends in order that the needs of vulnerable elderly people can be met at the time they and their relatives require. Professional help and guidance from statutory personnel or minimum hospital stay for diagnostic, medical, surgical or orthopaedic procedures, would be complementary parts of the total spectrum of provision.

Unfortunately, at present there is no such integrated approach to need. 'What the professional services can offer is a series of brief visits by specialists. What the old people need in addition – and sometimes more urgently – is extended contact' (Jones, 1972). Services vary from one part of the country to another. They tend to be patchy, very rarely provide a 24-hour service and demand that the elderly person fits them rather than responding to the needs of each individual.

Faced with these problems a variety of initiatives has developed in response, with the common objective of preventing institutional care. Some examples are the Hospitals at Home Scheme (Cang, 1977) and the emergence in a number of areas in the country of community care schemes, such as the Crossroads Care Attendants Scheme (Osborne, 1976). In these, caring aides are employed to provide help for vulnerable people who are unable to undertake tasks of daily living without help. Such schemes can complement services provided by statutory agencies and enable a package of care and support to be provided to meet individual situations.

SOURCES OF HELP

Mostly, frail elderly people have to take what the system decides is available to them and they are rarely asked about their preferences. The main sources of help are:

1. Family, friends and neighbours.
2. Health services – community.
3. Health services – hospital (Chapter 5).
4. Social and voluntary services (Chapter 6).

Family, friends and neighbours

Traditionally the family has always been regarded as the first link in the chain of support and there is frequently criticism that families, in our materialistic day and age, no longer take their responsibilities as seriously as they did in the past and are only too ready to shed them on to the welfare state. However, 'if our society is to see older people clearly in perspective, it is important that we do not clutter our thinking with out-moded myths and beliefs. The family of the recent past did not provide a universal harbour for its elders, despite the fact that what we now think of old age was fairly rare . . . The proportion of retired people is now twice as high as it was at the turn of the century' (Johnson, 1978).

Family structure has changed since Victorian times and gone are the days of large extended families. Today, it is the nuclear family which is the norm. Greater mobility of labour has meant that children frequently move away from the parents' neighbourhood, so that families have become geographically scattered and 'intimacy at a distance' has taken the place of daily face-to-face contact, links being maintained by car, the telephone and holidays together. An increasing number of elderly people from ethnic minorities face similar difficulties, for the role of the elder, which they would have expected to enjoy within the extended family in their country of origin, is denied them in our present-day society.

Living alone does not indicate family neglect. The inevitable result of a high birth rate at the beginning of this century and a very much lower one a generation later, has resulted in a number of elderly people surviving into later life without children or who have had children who have not survived.

Current situation

There is a growing number of very frail elderly people, many of them supported by a spouse equally frail or by ageing children, probably with children and grandchildren of their own and maybe facing the identity conflicts and the economic run-down of retirement. Strains on family life are increasing as witnessed by the number of divorces, separations and one-parent families. Yet evidence suggests that the majority of families shoulder the responsibilities of elderly parents without complaint.

Broad moralistic judgements about the duty of the young to look after the old no longer fit the demographic facts. It is acknowledged 'that most care in the community is provided not by formal services but by families and to a lesser extent friends and neighbours – often collectively referred to as "the informal sector of care" ' (DHSS, 1983). These informal carers are the front-line providers of support for 85 per cent of elderly people.

Where the elderly relative shares the family home, stresses can become unremitting particularly where problems of mental infirmity are involved. Clearly the implication of situations such as these is the requirement for resources both skilled and practical that elderly people and their families can call upon.

Services that are established by virtue of an Act of Parliament are called statutory services. The major users of the health and social services are elderly people and it is the very old and frail, those who either have the slenderest family resources to call upon or who lack relatives altogether, who make the largest demands.

Health services – community

Although various changes and reorganisations have taken place since the implementation of the NHS Act in 1948, the basic principle that the whole range of community health and hospital services should be available to any national of the United Kingdom remains.

Community health services have been in existence for some considerable time. However, the development of the *primary care team* (family doctor, district nurse, health visitor and their supporting staff make up the basic team) has provided an important stimulus to the expansion of domiciliary provision.

General practitioner service

For the majority of elderly people, the family doctor (general practitioner) is the first person he sees in time of illness and it is through him that the patient has access to any of the other health services he may require. Capitation fees for the family doctor's patients who are over the age of 65 are weighted and there is an additional increase for patients of 75 and over. This knowledge should help older people to feel less guilty about contacting their doctor. Frequently symptoms that earlier in life might have been considered important enough to seek medical attention are believed to be due to the ageing process and so remain unreported and untreated.

General practice has increasingly become group practice based on purpose-built premises which has the advantage that other members of the primary care team can be accommodated in the same building and this leads to better communication between all members. As already mentioned (Chapter 3) centralisation of premises and decline in home visiting can create problems for elderly patients. Alternative locations to group-practice premises are health centres where a number of additional facilities may be provided, such as chiropody, dietetic and, on occasions, community physiotherapy services. In inner-city areas which generally have a high proportion of elderly people, many doctors practise single-handed, relying heavily on deputising services and frequently without the help of the primary care team.

For many reasons general practitioners can vary in quality. However, examples of good practice, such as the provision of off-peak surgery hours, the establishment of well-elderly clinics and keeping a register of those in greatest need, are doing much to prevent illness and breakdown and inevitable admission to institutional care.

Community nursing service – district nursing service

In some health authorities, nurses are attached directly to doctors' practices and in others, as in the past, to a defined geographic area. Although attachment to a practice provides the satisfaction of working more closely with other members of the primary care team, it may mean increased time spent in travelling, since very few GP practices confine themselves to strict geographical limits. Qualified district nurses spend just under 50 per cent of their time with elderly patients and perform such skilled tasks as giving insulin injections, treating varicose ulcers, or, if there is a crisis of acute illness, they will attend to all nursing procedures. Nursing auxiliaries assist district nurses and give a great deal of simple general care and support such as bathing, dressing and undressing. A twilight service and, much less frequently, a night service is also provided by the district nursing service. Nursing equipment such as hoists, bedpans, special beds and bedding, can be provided through the community service often in conjunction with the Red Cross or social services to help elderly patients and their families at home. For people in the terminal stages of cancer, the Marie Curie Memorial Foundation provides nursing help during the night in some areas which can be a considerable support to the family involved.

Community psychiatric nursing service

The introduction of the psychiatric nurse into the community is relatively new. In the last 10 years or so the number of these nurses has increased rapidly and there are now more than 2000 working outside psychiatric hospitals. The role of the community psychiatric nurse is a varied one and involves giving practical help and advice and support to families, friends and neighbours on the management of problems of people with mental illness. In this way many can remain at home instead of having to be admitted to institutional care. The nurse liaises closely with the local psychiatric hospital and also with members of the primary care team, social services and voluntary personnel with whom she can act in a consultative manner giving specialised advice when required and back-up support.

Health visiting service

The health visitor's role is primarily concerned with prevention, the early detection of ill-health, and in health education. She has particular statutory responsibility for young children under the age of five and as a result only about 15 per cent of her time is spent with elderly people. Yet because of her specialised training a health visitor can be invaluable in identifying people at risk in the community and in providing help, advice and support.

Chiropody service

Chiropody is provided through the National Health Service to people in hospital and in the community. By far the largest group in the community is over the age of 65. As they grow older, people's need for foot care generally increases. Many find that because of physical incapacity or poor sight they are less able to care for their feet and as a result mobility is reduced and life may become increasingly circumscribed.

Chiropodists work in health centres or in separate premises. A domiciliary service is provided for people who are housebound or find great difficulty in getting about, and many residential homes for elderly people are visited regularly by a chiropodist. There are also growing numbers of mobile chiropody units which are helping to supplement services in isolated rural areas.

Unfortunately, there is a national shortage of qualified chiropodists and it has been estimated that only 1 in 6 of the elderly population requiring treatment actually receives it. In some health districts foot-care assistants, accountable to the qualified chiropodist, have been appointed, given appropriate in-service training, and are then able to provide a service for elderly people needing simple foot care, i.e. pedicure. Voluntary agencies, particularly Age Concern, are doing a great deal to supplement the service by assisting with finance, transport to near-by clinics and also providing a pedicure service at some clubs and day centres.

Community physiotherapy services

Since 1974, physiotherapy for patients in the community has slowly but steadily expanded and developed and is discussed in Part Two.

The effect of the Ministry of Health's statement in 1949 (RHB(49) 114; HMC(49)93) that 'the shortage of adequately trained physiotherapy personnel makes it imperative to concentrate them in hospital departments where their services can be employed to most advantage', did much to deter early initiative. Slowly, however, a few community physiotherapy schemes started to burgeon. The McMillan Report (1973), followed by a working party set up by the Chartered Society of Physiotherapy (CSP) (1973) to view current trends in community physiotherapy and the publication of the report *Physiotherapy in the Community* (Partridge and Warren, 1977) have, in conjunction with government emphasis on community care, given impetus to the development of the service.

Shortage of adequately trained physiotherapists still exists but the appointment of district physiotherapists has created opportunities to assess overall needs and priorities, so that resources can be reallocated to provide a more effective service and this includes the needs of patients in the community as well as those in hospital.

The development of community physiotherapy has particular advantage for elderly people. It is a means of offering a service that is, generally speaking, more sensitive to the individual needs of patients than that provided in an institutional setting. The use of at-risk registers and regular follow-up visits by community physiotherapists, following a patient's discharge from hospital, help to enable elderly people to maintain mobility and to provide support for relatives and others involved.

Community occupational therapy services

Approximately 20 per cent of practising occupational therapists work in the community and although in a few areas of the country these occupational therapists are health service based, the majority are employed by social services departments. Their role is discussed on page 76 and in Part Two.

REFERENCES

Cang, S. (1977). An alternative to hospital. *Lancet*, **i**, 742–3.
Chartered Society of Physiotherapy (1973). *Working Party Report on the Role of the Physiotherapist in the Community*. Chartered Society of Physiotherapy, London.
Comfort, A. (1977). *A Good Life*. Mitchell Beazley, London.
DHSS (1973). *The Remedial Professions* (McMillan Report). HMSO, London.
DHSS (1983). *Supporting the Informal Carers: List of Initiatives* (Report of the Social Services Development Group). HMSO, London.
Johnson, M. (1978). The good old days? *New Age*, Summer, 29.
Jones, K. (1972). *Easing the Restrictions on Ageing*, pp. 7–16. Age Concern England.
Osborne, P. (1976). *Coincidence or Meant To Be?* Crossroads Care Attendant Scheme Trust, Rugby.
Partridge, C. J. and Warren, M. D. (1977). *Physiotherapy in the Community*. Health Services Research Unit, University of Kent, Canterbury.

Chapter Five

HOSPITAL SERVICES

The popular belief still remains in many quarters that a high proportion of Britain's elderly population live either in hospital or in old people's homes. In practice, however, slightly over 94 per cent of people over retirement age live in private households. At any one time less than 3 per cent are in hospital and less than 3 per cent in residential accommodation. Nevertheless, the proportion of elderly people in both general and psychiatric hospitals makes heavy demands on available resources.

In 1977 some 111 000 beds were available to the four main hospital specialties of general medicine, general surgery, geriatric medicine and traumatic and orthopaedic surgery. While 67 per cent of those beds were occupied by patients aged 65 and over, 44 per cent of them contained patients of 75 and above (DHSS, 1981a). In psychiatric hospitals well over half the total number of patients are over the age of 65 and a growing proportion of these are people of 75 and over.

In recent years prevention of institutionalisation has been a major objective in planning services. This has been reflected in social service developments by the increase in domiciliary personnel and also in hospital policies, where growing emphasis is being placed on the diagnostic and treatment aspects of the service. As a result mean length of stay in hospital has steadily diminished. As through-put increases, so more patients can be accommodated. Laudable though such policies are, they have considerable implications for after-care and community services and on longer-stay hospital provision.

One possible answer to the latter is seen by central government to be the introduction of NHS Nursing Homes. As a result, experimental schemes have been set up in three health districts to test the practical implications of such a project (Hooper, 1983). Although some see this as a way of offering a better quality of life for elderly people than long-stay wards, others question whether the answer is to fill gaps in current resources with yet another type of institution rather than attempting to look at fresh solutions and a new pattern of overall service in the light of the changing demographic structure of our society (p. 50).

GERIATRIC MEDICINE

Trends in medical care have influenced policies in all hospital specialties including that of geriatric medicine where the aim over the last decade has been towards an acute high turnover and rehabilitation service 'away from asylum and long-stay care' (Rodgers, 1982).

Apart from the humane advantages to patients of shortened hospital stay, emphasis on these aspects has developed partly to highlight the need for acute facilities comparable with those of other clinical specialties and 'partly in a determined effort to change the depressing image of geriatric medicine in the eyes of the public, the medical profession and health administrators' (Exton-Smith and Evans, 1977). The reasons for the lack of facilities and the depressing image presented by the specialty lie in its history and development.

History and development

In 1834 the Poor Law Amendment Act established the workhouse as a means of providing for vagrants, the unemployed and the destitute, while workhouse infirmaries (often part of the same building) dealt with the sick and infirm. The principle adopted by each workhouse was that of 'less eligibility' by which no inmate could receive accommodation as good as that available to the lowest-paid worker. Little attempt was made to differentiate between applicants and the elderly and infirm, the mentally and physically disabled as well as the young and able-bodied were all crowded together.

During this period voluntary hospitals had been developing rapidly and these became centres of teaching and research. Since funds were limited, inevitably they became selective, preferring patients with acute illness to those who were chronically sick. This period also saw the creation of a range of specialist hospitals dealing with specific conditions and these included isolation hospitals and sanatoria built to accommodate those with infectious diseases and with tuberculosis. At the same period people with mental illness were incarcerated in vast asylums in isolated country places and then forgotten by society. By 1929 the Public Assistance Committees of the local authorities had taken over the management of the workhouses, apart from a number appropriated for use under the Public Health Acts. The latter gradually evolved into municipal hospitals, only very few of which were of a standard to equal the voluntary hospitals. In the majority, conditions were appalling and nursing staff minimal.

It was to such repositories of the chronic sick of all ages that pioneers such as Dr Marjory Warren were appointed in the 1930s and by their efforts gradually changed the negative image associated with these hospitals, with death the only outcome, to one of positivity and challenge. Bedfast patients were re-mobilised and several were enabled to return to the community. It took time, but it was shown to be possible.

The introduction of the National Health Service in 1948 led to a more equitable distribution of medical resources to meet the needs of a population of all ages. Some of the old Public Assistance institutions were taken over by the Health Service, many developing into the present district general hospitals, others remained with the local authority and were designated welfare homes. In recent years these have been replaced by purpose-built residential homes to accommodate a very much smaller number of residents.

Since 1948 and following DHSS policy, departments of geriatric medicine, based on district general hospitals, have been established in most areas of the United Kingdom following the example of the few pioneering departments developed in the 1930s. The function of these departments to which at least one physician of senior status is appointed is to provide a district service for people of 65 years of age and over.

Departments of geriatric medicine

The hospital beds on which the service is based were found in a wide variety of accommodation, such as upgraded workhouses, chronic sick hospitals, old isolation hospitals, sanatoria and small cottage hospitals. A large number of these buildings are part of the social history of our time. Although many of these hospitals have been closed, many still remain and the continued existence of poor accommodation tends to perpetuate traditional attitudes, namely that second-class buildings are all that is required for second-class patients. In spite of DHSS recommendations that a considerable proportion of a department of geriatric medicine's beds should be in the district general hospital, there is as yet no universal application of this principle.

On-site facilities for investigation, treatment and rehabilitation are frequently inadequate and geographical isolation of many of these units from the district general hospital and the mainstream of medicine can pose many problems. Discussion with colleagues in other specialties and access to the full range of clinical and remedial resources is difficult. Colleagues in their turn are denied the benefit of the department's advice and expertise over problems of management of their own elderly patients with particular 'geriatric features' (Burley, 1979).

This separation from other specialist services contributes to the widespread belief that the specialty is primarily concerned with long-stay back-up facilities for 'acute' services. A belief that is surely misplaced, for despite the fact that the majority of patients referred suffer from severe multiple disability and social disadvantage, it is estimated that over 80 per cent admitted to departments of geriatric medicine remain there for less than three months.

What is geriatric medicine?

The awkward word 'geriatric' derives from the Greek (*geras* = old; *iatrikos* = healing) and was first coined by an American physician, Dr Ignarz Nascher, in 1914 to denote the medical care of the elderly. To give the specialty of geriatric medicine a precise definition is difficult. Most specialties in medicine are identified on the basis of organs or systems of the body – cardiology or neurology, for example, or are based on therapeutic techniques such as surgery. Although geriatric medicine is concerned with elderly patients it does not, like paediatrics, deal with *all* the patients in that particular age-group, for patients referred to departments of geriatric medicine only make up a proportion of the total number of ill elderly people admitted to hospital.

'Both geriatric and general medicine are major users of hospital beds, both employ the skills of clinical medicine and therapeutics, and both manage patients with a wide range of illness' (Stout, 1979). What is the difference between general medicine and geriatric medicine and why do elderly people need their own medical specialty?

Special features of geriatric medicine

1. Age of patients referred

Although most hospital departments are increasingly affected by the growth in the population of the number of older people it is on departments of geriatric medicine that particular pressures fall. Currently three-quarters of the beds in these departments are occupied by patients over the age of 75 and it is this age-group that is most likely to have problems of a physical and psychological nature as well as of a social-environmental nature.

2. Specific characteristics of patients referred

Multiple pathology: Over the years multiple disease processes accumulate and in elderly patients, unlike younger ones, multiple pathology is frequently the main clinical characteristic. Patients referred are likely to be those whose precipitating illness occurs against a background of pre-existing disability, thus presenting complex diagnostic and later rehabilitation problems.

Altered reaction to illness: Illness frequently presents very differently in this age-group, with an absence of specific symptoms such as lack of pain in the myocardial infarction for example. As a result of alterations in pain mechanisms, pain sensitivity may be reduced. Body temperature mechanisms are frequently unstable and in consequence pyrexia, the expected response in an acute infection such as pneumonia, is often lacking. Alternatively, the sudden onset of transient confusion often replaces fever or other physical signs.

Reduction in drug tolerance: Absorption and excretion of drugs can alter with age, reducing the patient's tolerance to a wide range of drugs and producing adverse reactions as a result.

3. Other characteristics

In addition to the special characteristics of older patients a number of presenting symptoms of disease may occur. Named the 'Giants of Geriatrics' (Isaacs, 1980) these are:

IMMOBILITY – the inability to walk from chair or bed to and from the lavatory.

INSTABILITY – the tendency to recurrent and unpredictable falls.

INCONTINENCE – failure to retain urine or faeces, or both.

INTELLECTUAL IMPAIRMENT – loss of self-awareness of such severity as to render the individual incapable of self-care.

4. Social problems
No patient can avoid these, for in the treatment of disease each person must be accepted as a dimensional being and seen in relation to his psychological and environmental needs. Disability and loss of independence, problems of bereavement, economic hardship and poor housing all increase personal vulnerability. 'There are few pure social problems in old age. Breakdown is multifactorial and complex, requiring most careful analysis of all factors, both medical and social' (Brocklehurst, 1977).

Although there is frequently considerable overlap between the responsibilities of physicians in general and those in geriatric medicine, it is clear that very often more is required to meet the needs of elderly people for 'accurate assessment, personalised treatment, appropriate rehabilitation, comprehension of the social situation and the fine tuning of resources to abilities' (Isaacs, 1981) than can be encompassed by hospital-based acute medical practice.

As a result a comprehensive system of care and support has been developed, involving a range of skills and services in both hospital and community, known as geriatric medicine which is defined by the British Geriatrics Society as 'concerned with the clinical, social, preventive and remedial aspects of illness in the elderly'.

Organisation of departments of geriatric medicine
In general, departments of geriatric medicine seek to provide a service for a defined population (i.e. people of 65 and over) within the health district. Considerable variation exists between departments both in organisational terms and in criteria for admission. Most departments receive their patients as direct referrals from general practitioners. In-patient services are provided for those requiring acute admission and assessment, rehabilitation and continuing care. Services for patients at home include domiciliary visiting, out-patient services and day-hospital support.

Several developments have occurred over the years. Chief among these are the establishment of multidisciplinary teams and the organisation of case conferences; the emphasis on prevention and rehabilitation and the close links made with community personnel and primary care teams. For remedial personnel, the holistic approach to patient care; the need to visit patients in their home environments so that the impact of disability on daily life is seen in full perspective; the support provided by multidisciplinary team colleagues; and the opportunity given for personal responsibility, initiative and improvisation have for many staff become the only logical and satisfying way to undertake their professional work.

Day-hospital service

This service has no counterpart in general medicine. One of the main purposes of a day hospital is rehabilitation, and many elderly people's functional skills and mobility can be helped by attendance at a day hospital. Regular review is essential so that progress can be monitored and improvement maintained.

Although day hospitals are an important part of a department of geriatric medicine's service, difficulties have arisen over the years. Lack of adequate day-care facilities such as luncheon clubs, and particularly day centres, throw extra and often inappropriate demands on day hospitals (McNicholl and Comber, 1979). The increasing pressures on ambulance transport, the growing cost of the service (Hildick-Smith, 1984) and the tendency of day-hospital attendance to weaken the patient's link with his community services, are problems for which there are no easy answers.

The provision of a mobile day hospital or day centre in some areas and the shared use of day-hospital premises by health and social services staff in others are examples of ways in which local deficiencies can be overcome; open access to day-hospital services by general practitioners can do much to maintain the patient's link with his primary care team.

The future of geriatric medicine

In recent years a number of variations have emerged on the basic pattern of service organisation of the specialty. The increasing number of elderly people in other hospital departments has in some instances led to closer co-operation so that the skills of the department of geriatric medicine can be used to help in the management of elderly patients in other clinical specialties. One such example of co-operation has been undertaken in Edinburgh where the attachment of consultants in geriatric medicine and associated junior medical staff to acute medical wards to provide specialised help has resulted in a considerable reduction in the duration of the patient's hospital stay in acute beds (Burley, 1979).

In some departments of geriatric medicine physicians with a specialist interest in geriatric medicine have been appointed with responsibility for acute as well as geriatric medical practice. In others, age-related services have been developed in which all patients over a certain age including medical emergencies receive medical care from the department of geriatric medicine, while all patients under that age are accepted by the general medical department (Bagnall et al, 1977). Both these developments demand close co-operation between the specialties of general and geriatric medicine.

There has been much discussion regarding the future of geriatric medicine and the options available to it. With nearly 90 per cent of elderly people living at home, the gradual shift from an institutionalised to a community-orientated service with closer links with the primary care team, health, local authority and voluntary agencies would appear to have far more relevance for the needs of older people than 'old fashioned general medicine with its emphasis on episodic treatment and hospitals' (Williamson, 1979).

SPECIALIST SERVICES FOR THE PSYCHIATRY OF OLD AGE

Mental disturbance in old age is not a new problem, but because of the demographic changes that have taken place in society, particularly the dramatic expansion of the number of very elderly people, the proportion of those with psychiatric illness has increased considerably, so that the problem is very much greater. The needs of this particular group of elderly people together with the growing expectations from families, friends and neighbours for help with their care and support has led to mounting pressure on very limited resources.

There are many similarities between the development of services for the elderly mentally ill and the development of geriatric medicine. In each case specialism has occurred within a wider clinical field (i.e. general psychiatry and general medicine) to meet the requirements of elderly patients with particular needs.

Development of services

Like geriatric medicine, psychiatric services for elderly mentally ill people have undergone many frustrations over the years, not least the low priority given to their development. Although the need for such services is now generally accepted, negative attitudes to mental illness in elderly people and inadequate provision of resources in terms of finance, staffing and accommodation – mostly built at the turn of the century and frequently located far from main general hospitals – are some of the obstacles to progress.

Early development of these services relied very much on the drive and initiative of a number of pioneers, usually a psychiatrist, but in some instances a physician in geriatric medicine. More recently, government recommendations have stressed the need for health and social services to give priority to the development of services for certain priority groups. Among these are 'elderly people, especially the most vulnerable and frail and mentally ill people' (DHSS, 1981b).

Although specialist psychiatric services for elderly people with mental disturbance are being established in many health districts, not all as yet have this service. DHSS policy stresses the importance of creating in each health district in the country, local psychiatric services with accessible facilities to which should be appointed a consultant psychiatrist with a special interest in the psychiatry of old age.

At the same time, large isolated psychiatric hospitals 'near the end of their useful life' (DHSS, 1981b) are gradually being closed and it is hoped that the closures will release resources which can be used to develop new patterns of services, where possible community based, as an alternative to long-term institutional care. For, as the Health Advisory Service report *The Rising Tide* states, 'the problem is not just one for specialist psychiatric services which indeed only look after a small proportion of the more severely affected' (HAS, 1982). It also concerns other hospital specialist departments, community, statutory and voluntary agencies and the vast number of families and other informal helpers who undertake the major share of 'caring and coping' (Arie, 1979).

MENTAL DISTURBANCE IN OLD AGE

Because ageing is so frequently associated with inevitable physical and mental decline, mental illness in elderly people is invariably ascribed to irreversible brain disease or dementia, a term indiscriminately applied to a wide range of mental disorders in older age-groups, many of which are eminently treatable. Classification of these psychiatric disorders and the importance of accurate assessment and diagnosis are discussed in Part Two. Generally speaking 'mental disorder in old age falls into two major categories – dementia and depression' (Murphy, 1984).

Depression

Elderly people have many reasons for emotional disturbance and it is not surprising that depression is more likely to occur in this age-group than in any other. Although the majority of older people take life in their stride, some find it difficult to adjust to a changing world. Feelings of self-worth and personal value are slowly undermined by the loss of a fulfilling occupation, and for many, widowhood and death of contemporaries can mean increasing loneliness and isolation. Reduced income and status and loss of mobility and independence through handicapping disability are all factors associated with depressive illness in older people.

Much can be done by early identification and intervention to prevent severe depression. 'Sadly, it has been reported that 70 per cent of depressed elderly people are unknown to their family doctors, and older subjects are less likely to go to the doctor with psychological symptoms' (Murphy, 1984). Support and practical help during the process of bereavement, better social conditions, improvement in physical function and independence are all measures which can help.

Depressive illness can include a wide spectrum of emotional disturbances ranging from the reactive depression experienced in grief to more severe reactions including psychotic depression and the risk of suicide. Loss of appetite and of interest in the world around, difficulties in sleeping, self-neglect and restless behaviour and disorientation are all manifestations of a depressed individual. Most depressed people can be helped. In very severe cases admission to a psychiatric assessment unit may be necessary. For others anti-depressant drugs can be helpful although side-effects are frequently a problem. However, the most essential factor is continuing support and concern from family, friends and neighbours and the provision of adequate and effective community services, such as regular visits of a community psychiatric nurse or social worker, a home help and maybe attendance at a local day centre.

Chronic confusional state or dementia

The two main types of dementia from which elderly people may suffer are arteriosclerotic dementia, currently termed 'multi-infarct dementia' and senile dementia now known as 'Alzheimer's dementia' or 'Alzheimer's-type dementia'.

Multi-infarct dementia is responsible for approximately 12 to 20 per cent of elderly demented people; there is brain degeneration due to infarctions and impaired blood supply following a series of minor strokes with transient weakness in a limb and slurred speech. Improvement usually follows until the next incident and these incidents occur over a period of months with progressively less recovery on each occasion until ultimately mental function is seriously impaired. Progress is therefore intermittent and 'step-wise' in its development. Although not invariably so, patients with multi-infarct dementia frequently manifest signs of bilateral pyramidal involvement.

Alzheimer's dementia is the more common type and, unlike the step-wise progress of multi-infarct dementia, is characterised by a gradual but steady loss of brain function, invariably accompanied by senile plaques and neurofibrillary tangles throughout the brain's cortex.

Characteristics of dementia

Whatever the cause, dementia is characterised by progressive impairment of the higher brain function, leading to a deterioration in memory, in intellectual function and in social behaviour. However, except in late stages of deterioration some 'useful intelligence is retained and will continue to function if adequate time is allowed . . . Much confused behaviour becomes more intelligible if one sees it as a manifestation of anxiety – of the anxiety of people who can no longer rely on either capacity to deal appropriately with stimuli from the world around them or on the accessibility of their store of learned information. The world must be a very frightening place if one has lost these capacities . . . In these terms the repetitiveness of the confused can be seen as an expression of a wish for reassurance . . . of the need of people who are lost without their normal coping mechanisms' (Davidson, 1978).

Assessment

Mis-diagnosis of irreversible dementia can be a hazard because of the wide range of neurological, physical and psychiatric conditions which have very similar symptoms, particularly in the early stages of the disease. The first priority must be accurate diagnosis of this condition and the elimination of other remediable causes.

Management objectives

No drug treatment to date is available to halt or reverse the process of dementia and medication is limited to the relief of such symptoms as restlessness or behavioural disorders. However, the use of such preparations tends to make the individual drowsy during the day and wakeful at night thus causing a reversed sleep rhythm.

Essential objectives of treatment in its widest sense will be effective management of the person with dementia and support for all those concerned with his care. Except in very severe stages of this condition, and not all individuals go through this, the person's behaviour in normal social settings is likely to continue unchanged if he is not in a state of stress.

Dementia does not seriously affect habits and by controlling the environment by providing a normal social and physical setting and eliminating unexpected situations the individual with dementia can be helped to function in a habitual way. Skills that have been acquired during working years including a variety of simple household tasks can be encouraged. Not only do such activities provide purposeful occupation, interest and stimulus for the individual concerned, but they also do much to prevent such problems as behavioural disturbances, aimless wandering or restlessness at night. Much time and patience is required by those involved. Repetitive questions need to be dealt with sensibly and reassuringly and every opportunity taken to orientate the confused person to the reality of his surroundings. Impatience or failure to respond to the individual's demands for reassurance tend to exacerbate the situation and increase anxiety.

Such policies, however, do put tremendous demands upon those who are providing support in whatever situation they may be.

ORGANISATION AND OBJECTIVES OF PSYCHIATRIC SERVICES

Although there are a number of variations in the organisation of services for the psychiatry of old age, much depending upon 'population scatter between town and country' (HAS, 1982), the general objectives of these services will include the following criteria.

First, accurate assessment, either in the patient's own home, outpatient clinic or day hospital. Alternatively, assessment may be undertaken in the psychogeriatric unit or jointly with the department of geriatric medicine in the district general hospital. Assessment will be followed by diagnosis, identification of needs and appropriate treatment. Finally, continuing review and reassessment will be required together with continuing support for the patient and his carers, preferably and whenever possible in a community setting. If this cannot be achieved, residential accommodation, either in hospital or old people's homes, will need to be provided in as homely a setting as can be devised.

A multidisciplinary approach is essential together with collaboration with other hospital clinical departments, particularly with the department of geriatric medicine, so that a comprehensive service can be provided for patients with physical as well as mental disability.

Community-based support

Older people are happier at home and manage better in their own territory. Even those with dementia 'are secure in the reassurance of well-known cues, have the opportunity, and indeed the necessity to exercise the skills and abilities that remain to keep body and soul together and contribute to family life' (Stout and Tolley, 1981).

As already mentioned (p. 50) most care in the community is provided by families, friends and neighbours, but the stresses can be severe and much is required to relieve strain and provide professional help when needed. Adequate health and social services and close collaboration with voluntary agencies are essential in order that a network of help and support can be created to enable people to continue to cope.

Support from the primary care team, particularly the community psychiatric nurse; specialised help from the local psychogeriatric day hospital (including the very occasional mobile day hospital which can help to meet the needs of patients in rural areas) (Higgins, 1980); regular visits to a day centre run either by statutory or voluntary agencies, such as Age Concern in conjunction with MIND (Hobman, 1982); and the development of self-help and relatives' support groups are some of the resources available.

Residential care

Where mental illness is severe and for those without the support of family and friends, some kind of residential care will be required. If appropriate, residential accommodation may be provided in a local authority old people's home. Some local authorities have established specialist homes for elderly mentally infirm people and usually these will be visited on a regular basis by a consultant psychogeriatrician.

With the growth in private residential and nursing homes, the number of mentally frail people entering such homes is increasing. As discussed (p. 40), although these can be a valuable resource, measures to maintain standards are essential, as is the need to encourage 'adequate liaison between the private and the public sector' (HAS, 1982).

Long-term hospital support for people with mental illness puts tremendous demands on all personnel concerned in providing and sustaining some quality of life for elderly people in an institutional setting. Creating an environmemt, often in inappropriately designed buildings, which focuses on the individual and where patients are enabled to take part in a variety of interests that provide stimulus, preserve personal dignity and foster feelings of self-worth, takes time, energy and perseverance.

A continuing search is required for ways to help patients lead meaningful lives and to achieve and maintain their fullest physical and mental potential. Routines of daily living can be used as powerful therapeutic agents. In addition activities involving music, painting, gardening, for example, the use of reality-orientation therapy and the sharing of reminiscences of earlier days, recalled by the use of tape/slide programmes (*Recall*, 1982), are some of the means of helping patients to improve the quality of individual lifestyles.

Contact with the world outside the hospital, to establish opportunities for community involvement, multidisciplinary co-operation and peer support are a *sine qua non* if morale and enthusiasm are to be maintained.

Although mental disturbance is unlikely to pose a major threat to health in old age, the increasing proportion of people with age-related psychiatric disorders has put growing pressures on services which are still ill prepared to meet the needs of the elderly people concerned or their carers.

The two major categories of mental illness in people over the age of 65 are depression and dementia. Depression occurs most frequently in this age-group and much could be done to prevent severe depression by earlier identification and intervention and by improvements in individual physical health, social and environmental circumstances, and financial status.

Although demographic changes indicate that the numbers of people with irreversible dementia, particularly the very elderly, will increase over the remaining years of this century, a recent extensive study in Sweden and a small study in the United Kingdom reveal a fall in the number of elderly people with dementia, suggesting that an increase may not be so inevitable (*Läkartidningen*, 1983; Clarke et al, 1984).

REFERENCES

Arie, T. (1979). The psychiatric services: where do we stand? *Geriatric Medicine*, **4**, 54–6.

Bagnall, E. W. et al (1977). Geriatric medicine in Hull: a comprehensive service. *British Medical Journal*, **2**, 102–4.

Brocklehurst, J. C. (1977). In *Care of the Elderly*, pp 234–42 (jt eds Exton-Smith, A. N. and Evans, G. J.). Academic Press Inc (London) Ltd, London.

Burley, L. E. et al (1979). Contribution of geriatric medicine within acute medical wards. *British Medical Journal*, **2**, 90–2.

Clarke, M. et al (1984). The elderly at home: health and social status. *Health Trends*, **16**, 3–7.

Davidson, R. (1978). The problem of senile dementia. *Nursing Times*, **74**, 24, 932–3.

DHSS (1981a). *Report of a study on the respective roles of the general acute and geriatric sections of the elderly hospital patient*, p. 41. (Not published).

DHSS (1981b). *Care in Action. Handbook of Policies and Priorities for the Health and Personal Social Services in England.* HMSO, London.

Exton-Smith, A. N. and Evans, G. J. (eds) (1977). *Care of the Elderly.* Academic Press Inc (London) Ltd, London.

Health Advisory Service (1982). *The Rising Tide: Developing Services for Mental Illness in Old Age.* NHS Health Advisory Service, Sutton, Surrey.

Higgins, P. (1980). A mobile day unit. *Nursing Times*, **76**, 24, 102–4.

Hildick-Smith, M. (1984). Geriatric day hospitals – changing emphasis in costs. *Age and Ageing*, **13**, 2.

Hobman, D. (1982). Tackling mental infirmity in old age. *Remedial Therapist*, July 9th.

Hooper, J. (1983). An NHS home of their own. *Health and Social Service Journal*, pp 870–1.

Isaacs, B. (1980). Burden of care. *New Age*, Winter, 23–5.

Isaacs, B. (1981). In *Health Care of the Elderly*, pp 224–35 (ed Arie, T.). Croom Helm, London.

Läkartidningen (1983), **80**, 1079. (See *Therapy Weekly*, **10**, 29, 2. (9 February, 1984))

McNicholl, M. and Comber, S. (1979). Geriatric day hospital – remedial or social centre? *Physiotherapy*, **65**, 7, 210–11.

Murphy, E. (1984). Preventing mental illness. *Geriatric Medicine*, **14**, 2, 75–9.

Recall (1982). Help the Aged Education Department, London.

Rodgers, J. S. (1982). *Long-Stay Care for Elderly People: Its Continuing Evolution.* Oxford District Health Authority, Oxford.

Stout, R. W. (1979). Hospital care of the elderly. General or geriatric medicine? *Age and Ageing*, **8**, 3.

Stout, I. and Tolley, D. (1981). New knowledge about dementia. *Creative Medicine*, March, 35.

Williamson, J. (1979). Notes on the historical development of geriatric medicine as a medical specialty. *Age and Ageing*, **8**, 144.

Chapter Six

PERSONAL SOCIAL SERVICES AND VOLUNTARY SERVICES

Local government provides a range of services for elderly and disabled people through housing, education, social services departments and through a variety of other services and amenities. However, the level of provision varies considerably over the country and a great deal of inequality exists between one area and another.

Whereas health service costs are met, from taxation, by central government, services provided through local authorities are met mainly through local government funding, i.e. the rates. As a result the various departments such as social services are competing with one another for the limited funds available. The criteria for determining local priorities varies from area to area and it is unsatisfactory that elderly people receive help not so much according to their need but according to where they happen to live. It has indeed been said that it would be provident for every older person to have a Consumers' Guide before deciding where to live in retirement (Stevenson, 1981). For many no such choice is possible and at a time of economic stringency inadequate provision of social care hits hardest at the most vulnerable, among whom are the elderly and disabled people.

It is this group of citizens, the most disadvantaged, poorly housed on a low income, living on their own or with a marriage partner as elderly as themselves which puts the greatest demand on social services. As discussed, family networks, where available, continue to be an important source of support, but with an increasing number of very old people, the next generation of carers is also ageing.

The growing emphasis on care in the community is in line with the general disenchantment with institutional care and the wish of the majority of older people to stay in their own homes. However, this does have implications for domiciliary services both with regard to their adequacy and their flexibility in meeting individual needs.

As we know, pressures on informal carers are increasing and frequently there is little opportunity for relief from unremitting stress and strain. The present policies of 'high through-put' for hospital patients and discharge home before maximum functional ability has been achieved exacerbates demands on families and on social services. Innovatory ways in which to help people remain in their own homes are growing (p. 50) but many of these projects need guarantees of long-term financial support from hard pressed health and social services if they are to continue to develop. With reduced central government spending and competing demands on local government budgets, progress is unlikely to be rapid. So a great deal is required from social services departments to enable vulnerable people to maintain a satisfying life within their community.

LEGISLATIVE FRAMEWORK WITHIN WHICH SOCIAL SERVICES DEPARTMENTS MAKE SERVICES AVAILABLE

For many years there have been various Acts of Parliament related to the welfare of elderly and disabled people. In 1948 the National Assistance Act set out a series of welfare arrangements under different sections dealing with the needs of handicapped and older citizens.

In 1970 the Local Authority and Social Services Act brought together all these different services, placing responsibility for their administration and management under newly established social services departments, each headed by a director of social services and supervised by local councillors. This was followed in 1973 by the NHS Reorganisation Act (England and Wales) which placed statutory responsibility on local authorities to provide social work support for the Health Service.

Organisational patterns for social services departments vary. Functional models in which staff are responsible for particular services (e.g. domiciliary, residential or field services including health services) throughout the county, metropolitan districts or London boroughs are one way. Geographical patterns in which services are offered through local area offices with the aim of providing a more locally responsible service, are another.

Another important piece of legislation in 1970 was the Chronically Sick and Disabled Persons Act which reinforced the powers given to local authorities to help disabled and infirm people. With the passing of this comprehensive Act, it became the duty of the local authorities to identify the numbers of people living in their specific area who were substantially and permanently handicapped and to ensure that all handicapped people were informed of the services available to them. The Act also provides for the provision of welfare services including practical assistance in the home, TV and radio, assistance with travel, adaptations to the home, holidays, meals, telephones, etc.

The main responsibilities undertaken for the care and support of disabled and frail elderly people are as follows:

1. Assessment, advice and social work support.
2. Registration of disabled people. (This is a duty placed on social services departments by the passing of the Chronically Sick and Disabled Persons Act.)
   (a) The home help service
   (b) The provision of meals, including luncheon clubs
   (c) Incontinence laundry service
   (d) Night sitting service
   (e) The installation of telephones
   (f) Library services, including services for the special needs of the blind and partially sighted and the deaf.
3. The organisation of holiday schemes for elderly and disabled people.
4. The provision of day and work centres which provide social and occupational facilities and frequently a cooked mid-day meal.
5. The provision of funds and equipment for daily living and home adaptations.
6. The provision of residential accommodation.

Social worker's role

When an elderly person needs help, his first point of contact is usually the local office of his social services department.

The term 'social worker' describes people with widely differing levels of training and experience who are employed in a variety of settings. Because of the claims on qualified staff, particularly with regard to problem families and with chidren (for whom social work departments have a statutory responsibility), much social work with old people is done by less qualified workers called social work assistants. Although many of these have considerable experience and practical ability, pressures upon them are great and they have a great need for skilled support. In assessing the individual and his social situation, the social worker is usually confronted not only with the problems of a practical nature such as loss of independence in daily living activities, financial problems, etc, but also with those involving psychosocial and emotional needs.

Identifying problems, respecting the client's individual feelings and preferences are priority factors in the mobilisation of services and resources. Equally essential are such aspects as the difficulties of adjusting to disability, often a stroke, for example; the problems of inter-relationship when the older person is living with the family; or the effect of recent bereavement or a client's decision to enter a residential home. Sometimes if problems are chiefly concerned with the practical difficulties of loss of functional skills and mobility, or environmental limitations requiring reorganisation of the home, then an occupational therapist may make the initial visit.

Registration

When a disabled individual receives help from social services he is usually put on the handicapped person's register. In this way, local authorities can maintain their registers of disabled people living in the area. Disabled people are not obliged to register and a number of people, either from strong feelings of pride and independence or because they do not want to feel a burden, may refuse to be registered. However, being on the register as a handicapped person should not be regarded as a badge of disability but an indication that one is entitled to a variety of benefits as of right. It is in fact an administrative matter which in theory at least helps the local authority to estimate its future needs.

Occupational therapists

The majority of qualified occupational therapists working in the community are employed by social services departments to act as advisers on aids and adaptations for disabled people. Although many are attached to social work teams, organisational structures do vary in different parts of the country and in rural areas occupational therapists can be in very short supply indeed. Occupational therapists employed by social services are also involved in the organisation and supervision of work and day-care centre activities for elderly people attending day and work centres and for those in residential homes.

The occupational therapist visits clients at home to assess physical capabilities and to make recommendations to help the disabled person and his supporting family and friends. Such recommendations will include the appropriate aids required to help overcome problems of daily living and the type of adaptations needed to improve access to a bathroom and lavatory, for example, or to ensure adequate circulation space for a wheelchair user.

Good communication and co-operation with hospital-based occupational and physiotherapy colleagues, and also with community physiotherapists is a needful part of the community occupational therapist's role if a hospital patient's successful resettlement at home is to be achieved.

The home help service

The home help service which has been the responsibility of local authority social services departments since 1971, has expanded dramatically in the last 20 years. Not only does the home help give elderly, frail and disabled people much-needed help with the household chores and with shopping, but frequently the home help becomes the lifeline for the housebound. By the opportunity the home helps have to build up a close supportive relationship with many elderly people, they are able to keep a watchful eye on vulnerable situations and can report back to the home help organiser if help of a different nature is needed and thus have a crucial role to play in preventing crisis situations.

On average the home help visits twice a week during weekdays only, but if the situation is extremely critical, it may be possible to provide a daily service even including weekends. Many home helps in any case are providing a great deal of additional support for their elderly clients on an informal unofficial basis. Home helps are ultimately responsible to home help organisers who are usually based at social services departments. It is the home help organiser who visits the elderly person initially in order to assess the amount of domestic help that will be required and the amount the client will be charged.

Currently there are a number of anomalies in the charging policies of different local authorities. Some have a fixed charge, others have a means-tested charge, while some local authorities offer a free service. It is frequently said that the cost of individual client assessment and collection of charges can very nearly cancel out any income received.

Other home care and neighbourly services

A number of social services departments are extending the concept of the home help service to provide the same sort of practical support with the addition of some simple home nursing when required for elderly and disabled people during the unsocial hours not covered by traditional community services.

As a result there is a growing development of new forms of practical workers called variously care attendants or home care assistants, home aides, family aides and night sitters to help meet the problems of personal care encountered by elderly and disabled people living at home. Many of these workers receive a short induction training and in some cases training sessions from both health and social services.

As already mentioned, in many parts of the country a wide variety of schemes, some still in the experimental stage, is being initiated. Some schemes provide long-term continuing support for elderly and disabled people at risk in the community. A service such as a street warden scheme enables unobtrusive yet regular support and surveillance to be undertaken for vulnerable people in a particular area. Informal support networks within the community, such as 'patch-based' schemes which involve small local groups of statutory and voluntary workers or the re-allocation of resources from the statutory residential sector to provide alternative forms of help to maintain elderly people in their own homes, are just some of the innovatory forms of intervention now being developed (Kent County Council SSD, 1982).

Provision of meals

Approximately 50 million meals are served in people's homes, luncheon clubs and day centres annually. In spite of the fact that since 1962 local authorities were given the power to provide meals to people at home, the service is still very dependent upon voluntary bodies, particularly the WRVS. Meals are not generally provided at weekends, but if no relative is available a neighbour paid by the local social services department is often willing to cook a meal on Saturday and Sunday.

As with any type of blanket provision of service, there can be no catering for individual needs. The matter of choice, so vital where food is concerned, is eliminated as is the element of surprise, since the meals have a sameness and monotony that does little to encourage appetites and as a result meals can be wasted. Undoubtedly, one of the main advantages of the service to the elderly housebound is the opportunity for contact with meals-on-wheels staff.

Recent investigations have shown that the nutritional value of the meal is questionable since important vitamins are lost while the meal is in transit, that more sensitivity is required in meeting the needs of recipients from other cultures, and that elderly people themselves are too polite to express their true view (Johnson, 1982).

Luncheon clubs cater for more mobile people who are able to get out and about. Many older people lack the motivation for cooking a meal for one and cheap nutritious meals in these inflationary times are hard to come by. Luncheon clubs have the advantage of providing a main meal at a minimum charge as well as being a means of social contact. These clubs are usually run by voluntary associations and are assisted by subsidies from the local authority. In some cases, a certain amount of transport may be provided for the less mobile.

THE PROVISION OF AIDS, EQUIPMENT AND ADAPTATIONS

Much can be done to achieve maximum independence for disabled people by the provision of aids and adaptations that can reduce the handicap caused by disability.

Aids to daily living

Before an aid is provided careful assessment of functional needs must be undertaken so that the aid most suited to individual requirements will be supplied. It is equally important that having been provided with an aid the disabled person is taught how to use it and that any supporting relative or friend should understand its use.

Help and advice on the choice and suitability of a particular aid can be obtained from a number of sources which include the Disabled Living Foundation or from one of the growing number of Aid Centres situated in different parts of the country.

Many disabled people, particularly those who have lived with their disability for a number of years, have frequently worked out their own solution to a specific problem. As has been said . . . 'whatever people find helpful to reduce the handicapping effect of their disability can be described as an aid and it is only with the enlightened help of those professionally concerned and with the ingenuity of both professional and client that maximum independence will be achieved' (Fanshawe, 1978).

The supply of aids and equipment

The supply of aids and equipment for disabled people can be a complicated matter since frequently there is little clear-cut definition of responsibility between the different services involved. At the same time there is a good deal of variation in the system of supply between one part of the country and another.

In theory, aids which help activities of daily living should be supplied by local authority social services departments. Aids for nursing care should be supplied from the district health authority through the community nursing services. (The provision of wheelchairs is in quite a separate category and these are available through the artificial limb and appliance centres (ALAC) of the DHSS.)

It is sometimes difficult to determine whether an aid is to be used for nursing purposes or to assist personal independence. A commode, for example, could come under either category and it will depend very much on the individual situation and need. However, in many areas there has been little attempt on the part of both social services and health authorities to rationalise this service. In some parts of the country the situation has been remedied and guidelines have been formulated between the two authorities, agreeing which type of equipment is the responsibility of the health authority and which that of the social services department. In an increasing number of areas, joint stores of aids and equipment are being set up for the use of both the local district health authority and the social services department concerned and financial accountability allocated accordingly. Such arrangements do much to improve the efficiency of the service, but greater attention needs to be focused on more effective and less wasteful use of aids once provided, since it is known that a high proportion of clients do not use the equipment supplied.

Among alternatives to the present system, it has been suggested that disabled people should be able to choose their own aid with advice from professional personnel and an allowance from the government, a procedure followed by the majority of EEC countries.

Adaptations

For those living in privately owned accommodation, the Housing Act of 1974 made provision for local authorities to give improvement grants to help people who want to adapt their own homes. People in local authority housing usually have to undergo some financial assessment and to be prepared to make a contribution towards the cost of a major adaptation.

Some local authorities employ occupational therapy technicians who can make and install simple adaptations in the home on the recommendation of an occupational therapist. In some situations, particularly when someone is being discharged from hospital, the technician employed by the hospital occupational therapy department may be able to undertake the adaptation, in which case the department will be reimbursed by the social services. Use of a technician does help to speed up the process of getting the work done, which otherwise can take many months. Social services departments are also empowered to carry out adaptations to the home in order to help facilitate independent living for a disabled individual.

Adaptations can cover a wide range from quite simple features such as installing a second handrail on the stairs or altering the height of an electric power point so that it is more easily accessible, or widening a doorway for a wheelchair user, to new building such as a kitchen extension or a downstairs bathroom and lavatory.

THE PROVISION OF RESIDENTIAL CARE

The power to provide residential homes for vulnerable people is invested in local authorities by Part III of the National Assistance Act of 1948 (which is the reason why old people's homes are so frequently referred to as Part III accommodation). In the years that have passed since then considerable changes have taken place in the client group involved.

As a result of the demographic expansion of very elderly people, the average age of residents in old people's homes is now over 80 years and a very large proportion of these are physically and mentally frail. Demands on residential care staff have increased accordingly and although training opportunities have improved in recent years, there is generally insufficient emphasis on the need to encourage residents to maintain functional independence and mobility.

Whatever the reason, the decision to enter a residential home requires time, thought and discussion and when possible a preliminary visit to the home should be undertaken before final acceptance to meet staff and residents and get the feel of the place. It is important also that a person's own home is not given up until the initial period of adjustment is over in case he or she wishes to return home despite all its drawbacks. Such a policy, however, does not always occur and in situations of social emergency, immediate admission to an old people's home may be offered as the only solution.

The identification of people at risk in their community and the availability of appropriate advice and support at an earlier stage, for example in the case of the recently bereaved, does much to prevent such traumatic situations arising.

The objective of residential accommodation should be to provide an environment in which older people can live as normal a life as can be contrived in spite of disability and frailty and in which each resident's right to personal privacy, individuality, dignity and status can be maintained. For after all, the majority of residents up to the time of their admission to the home have regarded themselves as responsible adults capable of decision making, even if latterly requiring the help of others.

Unfortunately, the reality is often very different. Given a custodial and depersonalising environment, little opportunity for mental stimulus or for choice or decision making, segregation from the rest of the local community, and low expectations of clients' potential by staff concerned, it is easy to see why residential care is so frequently regarded as the end of the road with death the only way out.

However, this gloomy picture is not a universal one and a number of innovatory and creative approaches to new patterns of residential care have been developed in different areas of the country. Over the years there has been a shift away from the traditional model of an old people's home to the development of group living units in either purpose-designed new accommodation or adapted older buildings, so that elderly people can share communal facilities with a small group of other residents. Group living schemes of this nature are based on the concept of collective responsibility and can encourage meaningful relationships, give residents the opportunity to contribute towards the running of their own particular unit and undertake some of the domestic chores and simple cooking.

Residential homes are a community facility and there is a great need to break down barriers which exclude residents from ordinary life outside the home. Access to shops, church and local pub and involvement in community activities should all be available to residents if required. The use of the home as a venue for foot-care clinic, day centre, luncheon club or keep-fit organisation would provide a way in which residents could feel that they were helping to make their own contribution to community needs.

Closer integration between social services, health, housing and voluntary agencies in order to make the best use of limited resources and provide services that respond more closely to people's needs has already been discussed (p. 40).

In the case of residential care, such co-operation would have a number of advantages. For example, by using the skills and expertise of social work and health professionals, many residents of old people's homes could be socially and physically rehabilitated and enabled to return to live more independent and satisfying lives within their community. In this way residential homes would be used as a therapeutic resource rather than as a means of providing long-term institutional care.

Closer working relationships between health and social services staff would improve training opportunities for residential care personnel, by facilitating the organisation of more comprehensive and widely-based education programmes (Age Concern, 1983).

Finally, more imaginative links with housing agencies could enable the accommodation needs of elderly people to be met more flexibly. Short-term stay in a residential home could be used constructively, providing shelter and support for an elderly person during winter months and thus enabling him to cope in his own home on the return of the warmer weather; or perhaps providing alternative accommodation for him while housing adaptations, new building or rehousing were being organised to permit him to continue living independently in the community, summer and winter.

The private sector

Local authorities have recognised for some time that the major reason for admission to residential care is neither age nor disability but the lack of social support. As a result resources are being focused on extending domiciliary services rather than on increasing the number of places in residential care. In the current economic situation growth of services is restricted. Pressures such as the expansion in numbers of very elderly people and the greater need for after care for patients on hospital discharge have highlighted problems of supply and demand. A direct result of this situation has been the very rapid development in the number of private residential homes.

In the past, local authority old people's homes, together with a very much smaller but valuable contribution from homes run by voluntary agencies, have been the main providers of residential care in this country. Increasingly, however, the number of commercially-run homes is expanding, particularly in retirement areas in the South. By means of DHSS funding, they are being made available to many more elderly people than could have afforded such homes in the past.

Although commercially-run homes 'can provide high standards of accommodation and care' they can also provide 'the worst' (Johnson, 1983) and it is, therefore, appropriate that the Registered Homes Act 1984 includes detailed regulations for the registration of homes and a code of practice which will provide some control of standards and help to safeguard the needs of people in the private sector of residential care.

VOLUNTARY SERVICES

Voluntary effort is fundamental in the overall links in the support available to elderly people in the community, both at an individual level and by way of the many charitable and other organisations working in this field.

A simple definition of a voluntary organisation is one that is non-profit-making and non-statutory. Both central and local government have power to give grants to voluntary organisations and a number of services both local and national may be organised by the voluntary sector. Examples of this are the provision of services such as day centres and clubs, meals-on-wheels and luncheon clubs, home visiting, street warden schemes or the organisation and management of a national network of residential homes.

It is important to emphasise that voluntary organisations are not cheap alternatives to the statutory services. They have for many years played an important role in supplementing services provided by the statutory authorities, very often devising new and imaginative ways of meeting need and in providing help of a more personal kind. One of the most important functions of such organisations is to focus society's attention on areas of greatest need. With current limitations on public funding, the role of voluntary organisations is having even greater significance in bringing to the attention of both central and local government the importance of relating resources to such priority groups as the needs of people of 75 and over who represent the main growth area in our society.

Nationally there are vast numbers of voluntary organisations.

Some of these have been set up specially to help elderly people such as Age Concern England and Help the Aged, and many other organisations have particular relevance to the elderly and disabled. A select list of organisations will be found on pages 161–2.

REFERENCES

Age Concern England (1983). *Training Helpers in Caring for the Elderly*. Age Concern, Mitcham, Surrey

Fanshawe, E. (1978). Disability without handicap. *Nursing Times*, **74**, Supplement, 11.

Johnson, M. (1982). Meals on wheels up the wrong road. *New Age*, Winter, 20–1.

Johnson, M. (1983). Private lives. *Health and Social Service Journal*, July, 901–3.

Kent County Council Social Services Department (1982). Report of a Joint Working Group on *Services for Elderly People and their Families*.

Stevenson, O. (1981). In *Health Care for the Elderly*, pp 158–75 (ed Arie, T.). Croom Helm, London.

Part Two

THE ROLE OF THE PHYSIOTHERAPIST

INTRODUCTION

In Part One of this book some of the challenges and problems associated with ageing have been discussed.

Aspects described include the social and economic deprivation experienced by many older people with the loss of family members, of income and of status with retirement, and mention is made of the effects of ageing on body function and on the presentation of disease in later life. Attention has been drawn to the importance of recognising that the majority of elderly people live independent lives in the community or manage there with the support of relatives, friends and neighbours. At the same time it has been pointed out, that a number do suffer from physical and mental impairment and there is a great need for more adequate, flexible and cohesive services to provide skilled help and support for disabled people and the vast number of informal carers.

Rehabilitation, which developed largely in response to wartime emergencies, has had perforce to change its pattern as a result of the growing dominance of age-related disability and its interdependence with emotional, social and environmental problems of elderly people. Among current definitions of the term 'rehabilitation', one that approximates closely to the co-operative nature of the strategy required is that defined by Leonard Mayo in 1965 as 'A process of restoration, a practical and productive way of recognising the wholeness of Man and bringing to bear on his problems of illness and disability all of the pertinent knowledge and skills available. In this sense, rehabilitation cannot be claimed by any one profession for it belongs to many, nor by the professions alone for it belongs to the whole community.'

REFERENCE

Mayo, L. (1965). Cited in *Sociology and Rehabilitation*, p 208 (Sussman, M. D. (ed)). Washington, American Sociology Association.

Chapter Seven

THE ROLE OF THE PHYSIOTHERAPIST WITH ELDERLY PEOPLE

In discussing the role of the physiotherapist it is recognised that her contribution is only a part, although a very pertinent part, of the total knowledge and skills available.

The insatiable demands made on limited remedial therapy resources and the little likelihood of real improvement in levels of professional staffing, given the bleak economic situation, make it imperative that the role of the physiotherapist is an effective one and the service provided is responsive to the patient's individual situation, needs and wishes.

The majority of patients today suffer from chronic degenerative diseases which have one important characteristic in common, namely that their sequelae, a stroke for example or a lower limb amputation, have to be lived with since their underlying cause cannot be cured.

For physiotherapists this has meant a change in traditional styles of practice from acute crisis intervention, frequently undertaken with minimal inderdisciplinary consultation, to one of 'enablement in which a problem solving interaction between patient and therapist replaces the customary sequence of diagnostic assessment, prescription and administration of treatment' (CSP, 1983). This concept is fundamental to the professional role of the physiotherapist working with elderly patients. Table 7/1 shows a model of the problem-solving sequence of approach which has been designed by the Educational Development Unit for the Remedial Professions (EDURP) Working Party on the Care of the Elderly (1981).

Table 7/1 The problem solving sequence

6.	Evaluation of the whole procedure. (Accumulation of both conscious and tacit experience.)
5.	Skilled, continuing observation of the outcome of the therapeutic intervention. (Analysis of the effects of the therapy and the expectations.)
4.	*Action* (i.e. therapeutic intervention) by self or others.
3.	Decision making. Relating meanings based on observations with theoretical explanations/models resulting in a planned series of strategies for therapeutic intervention. The establishment of goals for the therapy.
2.	Ordering analysis of information concerning the patient/client's problem. Sorting out, and giving *meaning* to the observations.
1.	Collecting information. Skilled, informed awareness of events, signs, etc. (Possibly relying on an unconscious, tacit awareness of what to notice, and how to attend to it.) Sources: Referral notes, x-rays, case histories, patient report, etc. and examination.

Although the model has been set out diagrammatically in six sequential stages from assessment of the patient through to evaluation of the treatment plan, in clinical practice, however, the whole process is a continuum, in which the therapist has frequently to go backwards or forwards through the sequence.

For example, elderly patients usually present with a multiplicity of problems and the picture is seldom clear-cut, so that assessment is hardly ever a once-for-all procedure. Additional information, greater understanding of the patient's priority needs or social situation over a period of time, are among factors which may cause review and readjustment of initial strategies.

This ability to revise plans and accept the need to change 'is a key attribute of a good therapist, for only by critically reviewing the stages that have gone before is attention focused on particular needs, as opposted to providing an unthinking routine service. A professional as opposed to a technical task' (EDURP, 1981).

The physiotherapists who have contributed to this section of the book have indeed brought their 'pertinent knowledge and skills to bear on the problems of illness and disability'. While some have been concerned with a particular aspect of need, others have described the issues involved in the organisation, delivery and practice of hospital- or community-based physiotherapy services for elderly people.

Among aspects they have stressed are the following:

1. *The importance of critical assessment and the need for continuing review* because of the co-existence of disability and social and environmental factors. In addition to examining problems of physical function and understanding the social situation, assessment will frequently need to include environmental aspects of the patient's everyday living situation whether at home or on hospital ward as well as anthropometric requirements of furniture and equipment.

2. *The necessity not only of recording, but of pooling information* collected from assessment with all the other personnel concerned in planning the patient's treatment and management.

3. *The need to establish with the patient his priority requirements* and to set goals that are achievable and related to the practicalities of everyday living.

4. *The physiotherapist's ability to select and assign parts of the treatment plan* which can be 'done as well or even better by others' (Watts, 1971). In supervising, implementing and encouraging practice in self-help activities, remedial helpers, care assistants in residential accommodation, relatives and other informal supporters can have a major role to play.

5. *The need for evaluation of the outcome of treatment* so that its effectiveness can be measured and maximum use of scarce physiotherapy resources ensured. 'Such measures should not be the prerogative of researchers only, but become the daily responsibility of the individual clinician' (Bromley, 1983).

6. *The value of the multidisciplinary team* whose development requires a great deal of commitment from all the disciplines concerned. For the patient the interaction of people with a variety of skills and experience can ensure continuity of management and for individual team members, the team provides much needed support.

7. *The importance of education* both in regard to direct patient teaching and the opportunity it provides to indirectly influence patient care. Individualised education 'needs to outlast the physiotherapist's teaching, if it is to be effective. Evaluation of its effectiveness by measuring how much the patient learns, how faithfully he uses what he learns and what effect this seems to have on his comfort and function' (Watts, 1980) is an integral part of the treatment plan.

   The chance to influence patient care through indirect methods by working and advising professional staff in hospital or community should not be missed. Practical help and guidance for families and other carers on problems of management of disabled people and involvement in the training of non-professional personnel must be seen by physiotherapists as an important part of their role.

8. *The paramount necessity of establishing good communication* and regular exchange of information between all appropriate hospital and community personnel. Such action not only ensures continuity of management on hospital ward or in the community, but helps to avoid problems of hospital discharge and the patient's consequent failure to manage successfully at home.

9. *The needs of the physiotherapy staff* working with elderly patients with complex problems, frequently in peripheral hospitals away from the mainstream of medicine. Maintenance of morale by supportive senior members, the provision of opportunities to meet with peers and to update skills and knowledge by attendance at study days, seminars and post-registration courses, will help to maintain interest and commitment

10. *The importance of personal qualities of the physiotherapists* concerned, not only those involving professional competence, observational and critical abilities, but equally of attitudes. Problems of multiple pathology are regarded as a challenge to knowledge and expertise,

and the approach to patients is a positive one with the expectation of achievement.

Although the effort involved in encouraging motivation, helping to improve functional capability and restore confidence can take much time and endeavour, as against the easier alternative of disposal to long-stay care; for the patient concerned, there can be no comparison in terms of human dignity, self-respect and happiness.

REFERENCES

Bromley, A. I. (1983). Facts and fantasies. *Physiotherapy*, **69**, 11, 384–90.

Care of the Elderly, Course Aims and Topic Analysis (1981). Available from Education Development Unit for the Remedial Professions (EDURP), Albert Dock Hospital, Alnwick Road, London E16 3EZ.

Chartered Society of Physiotherapy (1983). Report of the Review Committee. *Physiotherapy*, **69**, 3, Supp 1–16.

Watts, N. T. (1971). Tank analysis and division of responsibility. *Physical Therapy*, **51**, 1.

Watts, N. T. (1980). *Patient and Family Education.* Lecture at the Annual Congress of the Chartered Society of Physiotherapy, Edinburgh 1980.

Chapter Eight

PHYSIOTHERAPY SERVICES IN A DEPARTMENT OF GERIATRIC MEDICINE

by A. Squires MCSP

The needs of patients referred to a department of geriatric medicine are almost always varied and complex, and as a result help will be required from a number of professional disciplines if treatment and successful management are to be achieved. These disciplines are usually those of medicine, nursing, rehabilitation and social work, with other professional departments providing specialised help as the need arises.

The ability of a department of geriatric medicine to provide a co-ordinated team approach to patients' needs, a high standard of care, an effective turnover and a conducive and supportive working environment for multidisciplinary personnel depends upon the close co-operation and imaginative and effective organisation of the professional services involved.

PHYSIOTHERAPY SERVICES

'Much has been written on the care of the elderly but little on the organisation of that care' (Hodkinson, 1983). The quality of the physiotherapy contribution to a department of geriatric medicine depends on many factors:

1. Attitudes of professional staff are central to the level of achievement of the service provided. Departments of geriatric medicine have the distinct advantage that the majority of physiotherapy staff involved have chosen to work in this specialty and consequently therapeutic optimism and positivity are the attitudes that prevail.

Multiple problems of elderly disabled people are seen as a challenge to rehabilitation skills and not as a reason for opting out.

2. Other qualities required will be those of patience and persistence since physiotherapists will encounter many delays and frustrations during the process of rehabilitation, particularly when arrangements for discharge have to be undertaken. It has frequently been observed that the patient and the illness are the easiest parts to manage and certainly there is no role here for those seeking quick results.
3. Pressures, however, are generally less than those experienced by physiotherapists working in 'acute' specialties, and there is time therefore to focus more adequately on patients' individual needs. As a result, successful hospital discharge can often be achieved and avoidable breakdown prevented.

WORKING AS A MEMBER OF A MULTIDISCIPLINARY TEAM

Membership of the team is frequently extensive, since patients' needs are multidimensional. In addition to the patient and his family, the team will include members from both hospital and community who are most able to provide appropriate help.

For the new member working as part of an integrated team, it is far from easy, particularly for those whose professional training provided few opportunities to co-operate with students of other disciplines. Initially at least, problems of professional identity, misunderstanding of the role of team colleagues and failure to co-ordinate efforts in achieving a common objective may occur.

With few exceptions there is little formal multidisciplinary education to date at student level (Beynon and Croker, 1983). However, a department of geriatric medicine can provide excellent opportunities for sharing knowledge, increasing understanding of interdisciplinary roles, and promoting and facilitating education and training for all staff allocated to the department.

Working alongside medical staff pre-and post-qualification, gives the physiotherapist opportunity to demonstrate skills and expertise to help medical colleagues to a better understanding of the therapeutic scope and limitations of physiotherapy and thus a greater appreciation of the importance of making appropriate referrals. With nursing staff, too, the foundations of co-operation should be laid during training, with regular physiotherapy contributions to classroom teaching and in practical help and demonstration on the ward.

Inclusion of the nurse in the team is essential if 24-hour continuity of patient management is to be maintained and individual functional independence encouraged. The introduction of the nursing process with its emphasis on patient- rather than task-orientated care will do much to reinforce these objectives and to 'help the development of the nurse's contribution to the team' (Mitchell, 1984).

The case conference

This is an ideal medium for the interchange of ideas between all disciplines. Traditional attitudes, particularly sometimes of medical staff, can be an inhibiting barrier to integrated professional co-operation. The case conference can provide a means of co-ordinating individual effort in working towards a common objective and creating a forum for two-way education and demonstration. In this situation therapists have a particular advantage in being able to demonstrate vividly *in vivo* or on video.

Leadership of the team

The successful functioning of the team depends on its leadership. Although it must be remembered that the medical member of the team has overall clinical responsibility, any member may lead in a particular situation or with a particular patient if the discipline concerned has the major contribution to make. In many instances the innovative medical consultant will vary the team leadership to encourage membership participation.

Team support

Not only is the team a means of achieving maximum patient care and management, it also provides a mutual support system for team members concerned with the very complex needs of elderly people.

Mutual multidisciplinary support can be particularly helpful in the event of a patient's death. All physiotherapists working with patients of an advanced age should be prepared to accept the frequency of deterioration and death. The decision to cease active therapeutic treatment while maintaining continuing support and the preservation of peace of mind and personal dignity will involve full team discussion. In this way feelings of anger and frustration at the expected demise of a well-loved patient can be brought out into the open and personal anxieties and feelings of failure examined and faced.

PRINCIPLES OF TREATMENT

The aim of physiotherapy treatment for older people is exactly similar to that for younger age-groups – to improve functional independence in order to achieve hospital discharge. Chronological age has little significance, save from the point of view of social history and the likely age of any relatives involved. Factors such as multiple pathology, atypical presentation of disease and the biological processes of ageing as they affect clinical practice should be considered and are well described in Payton and Poland (1983).

Assessment is the first priority and the sooner this can be undertaken and recorded, the sooner the team can meet to pool information and set realistic short- and long-term goals, essential for both the patient and the staff (Stewart, 1980), and plan and put into action the patient's individual programme of rehabilitation. Speed is important so that the hospital hazards of institutionalisation and dependency can be reduced to a minimum.

Review and reassessment will be a continuing commitment, to check and record change, modify goals where indicated and revise treatment programmes.

Records of individual patient assessment and treatment should be accurate and effective and available for reference. The problem oriented medical recording (POMR) system of notekeeping (Heath, 1978) is particularly appropriate for use in a department of geriatric medicine, because of the emphasis on problem solving.

Priorities for treatment usually have to be established because of staffing limitations. As a result, a system of priorities based on anticipated therapeutic outcome needs to be developed and in order to be cost-effective the major proportion of qualified physiotherapy time will be concerned with patients most likely to respond to treatment. Technology should be considered to complement physical treatments; biofeedback (Caudrey and Seeger, 1981) and video (Barefoot, 1983; Robson, 1981) are of particular interest to therapists.

Slower-stream patients will also require help, particularly in maintaining maximum physical function in order that some degree of personal independence can be encouraged, to improve quality of life and to prevent greater dependency on nursing staff. It has been reported that 24 per cent of patients who were in hospital longer than a year were discharged the ensuing year (Hodkinson, 1983), and so the labelling of patients as 'long-stay' needs to be undertaken with care.

Teaching skills are an important part of physiotherapy practice, not only in improving patients' functional skills but in providing advice and training for all those concerned with the patients' management and support. In this way appropriate parts of the treatment programme such as supervising chair drill, walking practice or stair climbing can be allocated to other members of the team, including trained remedial helpers, nursing staff, relatives and volunteers (Brocklehurst and Shergold, 1969).

The treatment venue

A well-appointed physiotherapy department has many advantages, but these have to be weighed against the undoubted disadvantages of time-consuming transportation of patients to and from the ward and the loss of opportunity to involve nursing staff in the principles and practice of individual patient handling and management. Whenever possible and practical, it is good that treatment should be undertaken in both ward and department so that all rehabilitation needs can be met.

Hospital discharge

The length of a patient's hospital stay in a department of geriatric medicine has fallen from an average of 109 days in 1972 to 77 days in 1979, while 50 per cent of patients are discharged within 20 days (DHSS, 1982). It is crucial for successful return to the community, and resettlement there, that the patient's hospital discharge is carefully planned by all concerned, so that inappropriate decisions such as a last-minute referral for 'functional assessment' or discharge home when statutory personnel are least available, are avoided. The distress caused for patient and supporters by unsuccessful discharge and re-admission is a hard and sobering lesson for all staff concerned. A survey by Graham and Livesley (1983) showed that the highest rate of early re-admission was due to inadequate rehabilitation – mainly where the advice of remedial staff had been disregarded.

Planning for resettlement in the community is a complex exercise, involving continuous and regular discussion not only between patient and relative and hospital team, but also with the primary care team, social services personnel, and particularly the home help involved.

Visits to the patient's home or to residential accommodation with occupational therapy colleagues prior to discharge, are essential to define problems and to give advice to relatives or care attendant staff on how best to help and encourage elderly people to maintain independence and mobility.

A trial visit home for a few days can help the patient to establish confidence in personal ability before final discharge; similarly, a few visits to the day hospital from the ward will allow the patient to become familiar with a new environment and unfamiliar staff before regular attendance, after settlement at home.

Successful maintenance in the community will depend on the adequacy of support provided both on an informal basis from friends and neighbours and by statutory and voluntary agencies. Regular follow-up visits by the hospital or community physiotherapist may be necessary until the individual's ability to manage has been established.

STAFFING REQUIREMENTS

Organisation and deployment

The suggested staffing requirements of a 250-bedded department of geriatric medicine concerned with patients with acute, rehabilitative and long-stay are as follows (BMA, 1976):

Physiotherapists	5
Occupational therapists	6
Remedial helpers	11

However, much will depend on the following:

1. Staffing levels will be influenced not only by the overall organisation of the district's physiotherapy resources and the priority given to the needs of elderly people, but also by the policy of individual departments of geriatric medicine concerned. If the focus is on rehabilitation and on reducing to a minimum the length of hospital stay, an adequate allocation of remedial therapy will be essential. If a day hospital is provided then an appropriate number of therapy personnel will be required for this service.
2. A department of geriatric medicine's physiotherapy staff may well be concerned in providing expert help in a number of places and these too must be taken into account when considering staffing requirements. Such situations will include physiotherapy advice

and guidance to elderly people and their supporters at home or in residential accommodation; attendance at the department's medical out-patient clinic to give help on mobility problems; or the giving of specific assistance to colleagues working with elderly patients in medical or orthopaedic wards.

3. Although the physical resources of departments of geriatric medicine have improved over the years, beds still tend to be geographically scattered. Problems of staff deployment, of transport and of the maintenance of staff morale in outlying isolated hospitals are not easily overcome. Trained remedial helpers, who may have the advantage of living locally, can make a valuable contribution, given regular supervision and support by qualified remedial therapists.

NEEDS OF STUDENTS AND NEWLY QUALIFIED PHYSIOTHERAPISTS

The consequences of an ageing population mean that all remedial therapy staff, with few exceptions, will spend the greater part of their professional time working with patients of an advanced age. The quality of the service they provide will depend on the standard and relevance of the training and experience they have undergone.

Physiotherapy students and recently qualified staff allocated to a department of geriatric medicine frequently have considerable anxiety about working with elderly people. There is a tendency to think that nothing new will be learned, that the problems of older patients are unrewarding and insoluble, that treatments will be of doubtful value and that the pace will be slow and frustrating.

The objectives for allocated students and staff should ensure that at the end of the allocation, the following principles will be learned:

1. The importance of accurate assessment because of the complexities of multiple pathology.
2. The need to adapt treatment techniques to meet patients' many medical and social requirements.
3. The importance of an integrated multidisciplinary approach to treatment and management and to resettlement in the community.

Exposure of students in training to elderly patients in a department of geriatric medicine may have been inadequate and frustrating for a number of recently qualified staff. It is, therefore, imperative that a programme should be planned that is both rewarding and imaginative, giving opportunities for staff to acquire greater knowledge and understanding of the needs of elderly disabled people and to improve skills and expertise.

Such allocated staff should be included in ward rounds, case conferences, home assessment visits and in regular teaching sessions; they should be encouraged to contribute to the departments' work from their own fresh viewpoint and recently acquired knowledge. Working with an experienced senior physiotherapist, newly qualified staff and students can undertake responsibility for patients according to individual experience and capability and, working together with team colleagues, will be accountable for their patients' progress.

De-briefing at the completion of this kind of allocation frequently demonstrates a total reversal of previous attitudes. Although many physiotherapists will still not choose to make a career in the specialty of geriatric medicine, a number will in time do so.

Support of physiotherapy personnel

With the establishment of an effective department of geriatric medicine, the needs of staff are sometimes overlooked. In general, physiotherapists have a high job satisfaction: staff groupings are small and manageable, and there is considerable personal autonomy with a high ratio of patients (Attwood, 1983). However, in such a situation constant vigilance by the physiotherapy manager is required. Although the rehabilitation of elderly people is a rewarding experience, it is seldom straightforward. Results come slowly and it can be difficult on occasions to maintain morale and positivity. It is essential that opportunities are made available for staff to update skills and knowledge by attending post-registration courses, study days and seminars. A continuing training programme for remedial helpers, combined with visits to local day centres, residential homes or an aids centre, for example, will increase understanding and help to retain interest and enthusiasm (Age Concern, 1983).

DEPARTMENTAL MANAGEMENT

The superintendent physiotherapist in such a department will require a wide range of personal qualities, together with the ability to organise, deploy and support staff; to co-ordinate activities of multidisciplinary personnel; to be involved in the planning and design of the patients' environment in order to maximise opportunity for remedial activity; and finally to have an extensive knowledge of the role and practice of geriatric medicine, the needs of patients referred and the local community resources available.

Peer support is essential as is multidisciplinary effectiveness both at ward and at management level. The multidisciplinary management team can be a valuable forum for department heads and should be encouraged.

SUMMARY

Multidisciplinary teams are essential, but complex, and need to be nurtured. The physiotherapy contribution will vary, but assessment, realistic aims and the sharing of activities wherever possible, are essential requirements. Students of all disciplines have an ideal environment in a department of geriatric medicine in which to practise teamwork and to learn the skills required to meet the needs of the age-group of patients with whom they will become increasingly involved once qualified.

The future of geriatric medicine can only be viewed as progressive and exciting when its importance in the health care of the whole population is realised. Finally, the essential ingredient for any member of a department of geriatric medicine is a sense of humour. The stresses, disappointments and frustrations can be overcome if the staff of all disciplines can laugh together.

REFERENCES

Age Concern England (1983). *Training Helpers in Caring for the Elderly*. Age Concern, Mitcham, Surrey.

Attwood, C. A. and Woolf, D. A. (1982). Job satisfaction of physical therapists. *Health Care Management Review*, 7, 1, 81–6.

Barefoot, C. (1983). Video – an aid for the '80s. *Occupational Therapy*, **46**, 9, 260–1.

Beynon, G. P. J. and Croker, J. (1983). Multidisciplinary education in geriatric medicine. *Age and Ageing*, **12**, Supplement, 26–9.

Brocklehurst, J. and Shergold, M. (1969). Old people leaving hospital. *Gerontilogia Clinica*, **2**, 115–26.

Care of the Elderly (1976). British Medical Association, London.

Caudrey, D. J. and Seeger, B. R. (1981). Biofeedback devices as an adjunct to physiotherapy. *Physiotherapy*, **67**, 12, 371–6.

DHSS and Office of Population, Censuses and Surveys (1982). *Hospital In-Patient Enquiry: Summary Tables 1979*. HMSO, London.

Graham, H. and Livesley, B. (1983). Can readmissions to a geriatric medical unit be prevented? *Lancet*, **1**, 404–6.

Heath, J. R. (1978). Problem oriented medical systems. *Physiotherapy*, **64**, 9, 269–70.

Hodkinson, H. M. (1983). *Long-term care*. Harrogate Seminar Report 7 – Effective Geriatric Medicine. HMSO, London.

Mitchell, J. R. A. (1984). Is nursing any business of doctors? A simple guide to the nursing process. *British Medical Journal*, **288**, 216–21.

Payton, O. and Poland, J. (1983). Ageing process. Implications for clinical practice. *Physical Therapy*, **63**, 1, 41–8.

Robson, P. (1981). Day/night communication in a geriatric hospital. *Age and Ageing*, **10**, 1, 60–1.

Stewart, C. (1980). A prediction score for geriatric rehabilitation prospects. *Rheumatology and Rehabilitation*, **19**, 239–45.

FURTHER READING

British Geriatric Society and the Royal College of Nursing (1975). *Improving Geriatric Care in Hospitals*. Whitefriars Press, London.

Brocklehurst, J., Andrews, K., Richards, B. and Laycock, P. (1978). How much physical therapy for patients with stroke? *British Medical Journal*, **1**, 1307–10.

Coakely, D. (ed) (1982). *Establishing a Geriatric Service*. Croom Helm, London.

Edelwich, J. and Brodsky, A. (1980). *Burnout: Stages of Disillusionment in the Helping Professions*. Human Sciences Press, London.

Geriatrics, I and II (1976). *Physiotherapy*, **62**, 5, 145–59; and 6, 178–84.

The Organisation of the In-Patient's Day (1976). HMSO, London.

The Oswestry Standing Frame (letter) (1983). *Physiotherapy*, **69**, 4, 129.

Ransome, H. (1978). Rehabilitation principles applied to physiotherapy for the elderly. In *An Ageing Population* (ed Carver, V. and Liddiard, P .). Hodder and Stoughton, London.

Sainsbury, R. and Mulley, G. P. (1982). Walking sticks used by the elderly. *British Medical Journal*, **284**, 1751.

Sim, J. (1983). Ethical considerations in physiotherapy. *Physiotherapy*, **69**, 4, 119–20.

Speck, P. and Ainsworth-Smith, I. (1982). *Letting Go: Caring for the Dying and Bereaved*. SPCK, London.

Squires, A. J. (1983). Using the tilt table for elderly patients. *Physiotherapy*, **69**, 5, 150–2.

Squires, A. and Livesley, B. (1984). Beware of burnout. *Physiotherapy*, **70**, 6, 235–8.

Ward, D. (1980). Setting up a physiotherapy service in a psychiatric hospital. *Physiotherapy*, **66**, 12, 401–2.

Chapter Nine

PSYCHOGERIATRICS

by J. Priest MCSP, DipTP

Although the psychiatry of older people has a great deal in common with that of younger age-groups, negative attitudes towards ageing and illness, particularly mental illness, have meant that there has been little effort in the past to provide an exact diagnosis and a planned approach to individual management. The elderly patient has been classed as 'demented' or 'senile' and thus only fit for disposal to some form of institutional care.

It is only in the last 20 years that psychogeriatrics has developed as a branch of psychiatry concerned with the total range of psychiatric disorders occurring in people over the age of 65. There are now growing numbers of consultant psychiatrists with special responsibility for the accurate assessment, diagnosis and management of elderly people suffering from psychological problems.

The word *accurate* is important because:

(a) many physical illnesses can manifest themselves as psychological disorders, and

(b) many psychiatric conditions, if correctly diagnosed, can be successfully treated, or, alternatively, symptoms alleviated, thus enabling people to live as fully as possible.

ELDERLY MENTALLY ILL

Although the word 'psychogeriatric' is often used to describe elderly patients with psychiatric disorders, replacement by the more appropriate and less denigratory term 'elderly mentally ill' should always be encouraged, since this implies that although elderly the individual is ill and therefore can be helped and frequently cured.

Mental and physical aspects of illness

Because of the close interrelationship (Fig. 9/1) between physical and mental illness in elderly people, improvement in one usually means improvement in the other. Physical ill-health in elderly people may

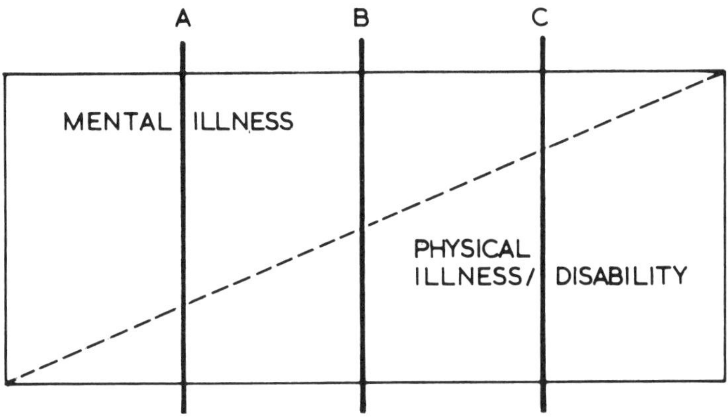

Fig. 9/1 The interrelationship between the mental and physical aspects of illness. All three patients A, B, and C could produce some degree of mental symptoms; 'A' has a severe mental illness but only minor physical disability; 'B' has a moderate amount of both mental and physical illness; 'C' has a very mild degree of mental illness but a very severe physical disability (Courtesy of Bergmann, K. (1972). *The Aged: Their Understanding and Care.* Stellar Press, Hatfield.)

aggravate mental illness and a person with mild dementia, for example, who develops an infection frequently experiences an exacerbation of his mental symptoms. Alternatively, a sudden confusional state, rather than a high temperature, can be a manifestation of pneumonia in an older person. Once the pneumonia is treated, behaviour will return to the pre-illness state.

Classification of psychiatric disorders in elderly people (Fig. 9/2)

Identification of the psychiatric illness will provide guidance in the nature and likely development of the disorder. However, diagnosis

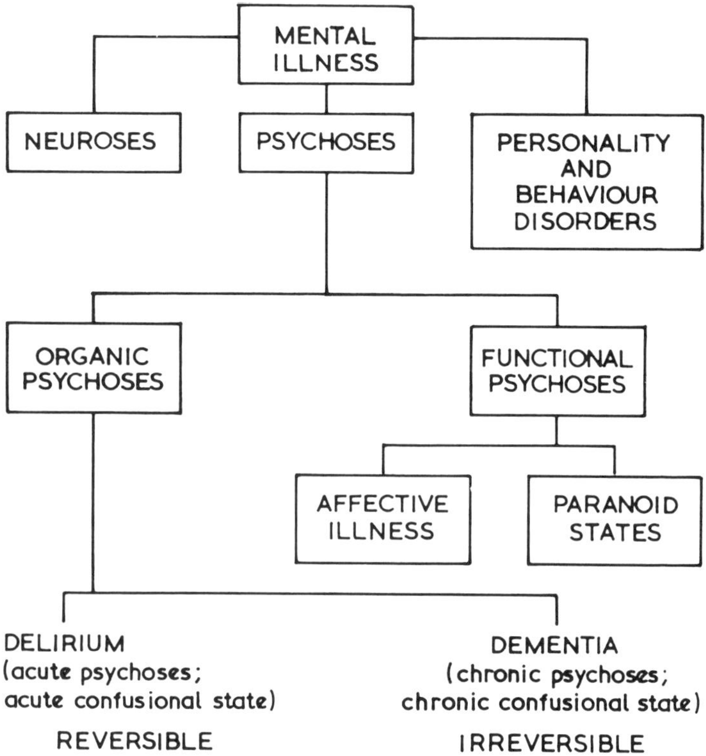

Fig. 9/2 Classification of psychiatric disorders in elderly people

will involve a great deal more than this if effective management is to be achieved. Older people can suffer from many pathologies and the majority have been exposed throughout their life to all kinds of emotional and social stresses and strains. Reactions to problems differ enormously between one individual and the next for, as Dr Bruce Pitt (1976) has said 'personality is paramount, colouring the clinical picture and materially modifying the outcome'.

Causes of delirium

D —	Drugs (uncontrolled or incorrectly administered) barbiturates, tranquillisers, alcohol Discomfort – constipation, urinary retention	
E —	Emergencies	Accidents, e.g. concussion (head injury), subdural haematoma, any anaesthetics or operations, e.g. fractured neck of femur Psychological, e.g. change of circumstances (bereavement), change of surroundings (hospitalisation)
L —	Less oxygen or blood to the brain, e.g. respiratory failure, stroke, heart failure	
I —	Infection – pneumonia, genito-urinary. pulmonary tuberculosis	
R —	Renal failure	
I —	Infarction – cerebral, cardiac, pulmonary	
U —	Unidentified causes, e.g. cancer	
M —	Metabolic, e.g. myxoedema, diabetes, uraemia	

Causes of the dementias

D	—	Demyelinating causes, e.g. multiple sclerosis
E	—	Early pre-senile dementias, e.g. Alzheimer's disease, Pick's disease, Jacob-Creutzfeld disease
M	—	Metabolic causes, e.g. myxoedema
E	—	Encephalopathies, e.g. Wilson's disease, alcohol, chemicals, vitamin deficiencies, metals, e.g. aluminium
N	—	Nutritional, e.g. avitaminosis (vitamin B complex), malnutrition, malabsorption (pernicious anaemia)
T	—	Toxic – alcohol Tumours
I	—	Infection – (bacterial or viral), neurosyphilis (GPI)
A	—	Arteriosclerotic dementia (now called multi-infarct dementia (MID))
S	—	Senile dementia of the Alzheimer type (SDAT)

The aim today is to enable older people to remain at home within their own environment. Admission to hospital should be avoided whenever possible as a change in environment can be disastrous for a person suffering a mental illness. Help may be needed from the community services in order to achieve this. It is very important to build up community facilities in order to give the necessary support to those friends and families who are caring for the mentally ill in the community.

Patients come from a variety of sources, e.g. from hospital departments of psychiatry and geriatric medicine, from the community, from residential accommodation and so on. Some have grown old in mental hospitals (the so-called 'graduates'). Many such people need no longer be in hospital either because the illness is well controlled by medication or has 'burnt itself out'. There will, however, still be a very small proportion of vulnerable people who in spite of adequate community facilities will need long-term support in some kind of sheltered environment.

PHYSIOTHERAPY

Whether physiotherapy is given in a department within a large psychiatric hospital, or in a psychiatric unit within a general hospital,

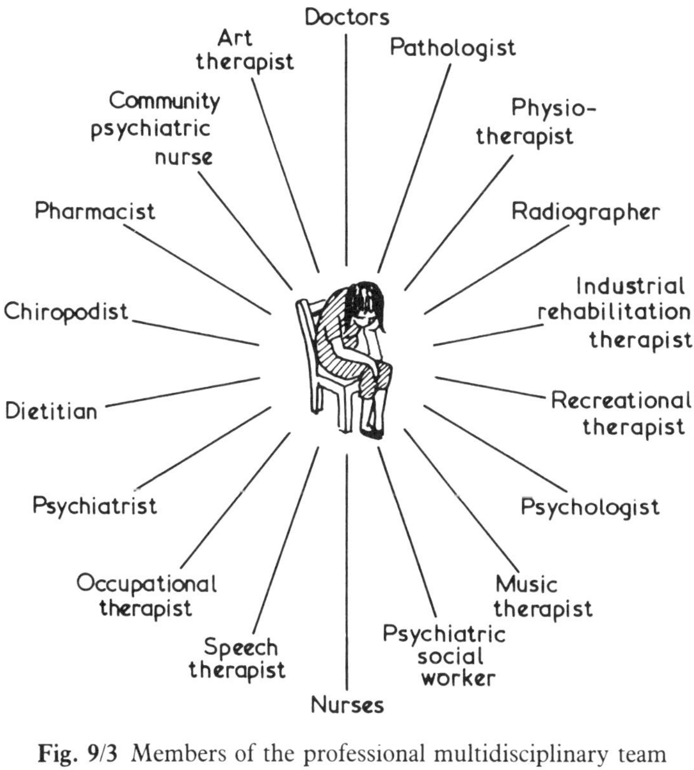

Fig. 9/3 Members of the professional multidisciplinary team

the basic objective is the same, namely to achieve independence. In this aim the physiotherapist will be part of a team (Fig. 9/3). The various physiotherapeutic techniques do not differ from those used in general hospitals. However, although the whole person approach is the principle underlying all physiotherapy in this specialty, the physiotherapist is very much more aware of the importance of the mental state and its influence upon the physical aspect.

The role of the physiotherapist can be divided into *four* categories:

1. Assessment
2. Clinical
3. Advisory
4. Educational

Assessment

As mentioned already, until recently anyone over 65 requiring treatment for a mental illness or entering a mental hospital tended to be labelled 'senile' implying failure of body and mind. This label remained for life, with the person having little chance of ever leaving hospital. It is vitally important this does not occur again and to this end assessment is crucial.

Assessment can take place over several weeks so that the psychological, physical and social aspects can be investigated fully. Physiotherapists need to:

1. Discover the patient's potential.
2. Prevent any physical and mental deterioration.
3. Increase or maintain the patient's level of independence.
4. Develop and practise skills (i.e. activities of daily living, etc).
5. Set both short- and long-term goals.

It is important that there is close involvement and co-operation between all members of the multidisciplinary team to achieve the proposed goals. Reassessments must be done frequently so that the patient's progress can be noted and goals reset and modified according to the current situation. Treatment depends upon assessment.

Clinical

It must be remembered that the patient has two conditions, the physical and the psychiatric. It is the physical condition which is the main concern of the physiotherapist, but she needs to be aware of the psychiatric condition as well. Treatment can be given on an individual basis or within a group depending upon circumstances.

Individual treatment

Retraining mobility

A very important aspect of physiotherapy is the retraining of mobility. Many patients literally 'go off their feet' even after an illness of one or two days' duration. Some tend to lose awareness of the vertical posture so that they tend to walk 10–15° off centre, either backwards or sideways. It is as if the 'centre' for controlling vertical posture is somehow set out of true. In some this can be 're-set' by getting patients to lie prone for 15–20 minutes daily, or by the use of a tilt table, or balance exercises in front of a mirror in order to gain the necessary postural adjustments.

As well as improving or maintaining mobility, prevention of contractures is another important aspect of a physiotherapist's work. Those joints which are at risk of stiffening must be put through a full range of movements if possible. This must be carried out regularly and can be done passively, or actively, depending upon the patient's tolerance.

Retraining mobility may necessitate proceeding through all the various stages from lying, sitting and standing, prior to walking re-education. The correct use of walking aids such as frames and sticks must be taught. Care must be taken in the selection of aids as aggressive or disturbed patients may use them as weapons to trip or injure people.

Physiotherapists must be aware of what is normal and abnormal in walking patterns, as many patients exhibit unusual patterns. Consideration must be given to such questions as:

1. Was the patient's gait normal prior to his illness?
2. Is the abnormal gait the result of a neurological condition, or the result of medication?
3. Is the unusual gait a result of the psychiatric condition? (Are the 'voices' telling the patient to walk as he is?)

The problems must be identified before treatment can be effective.

It is also important to remember that the patient may have an altered pain response so that pain is not appreciated, or may be more easily forgotten, or accepted, or may generally be less severe. It is not unknown for an agitated and confused patient to walk with a fractured femur.

Once the patient is ambulant, regular walks to the lavatory will help to maintain confidence. Here the co-operation of the nursing staff is of prime importance. Lavatories can be made easier to recognise by the addition of labels, or by having the doors painted a bright colour. Once mobile, the patient should be taught to use stairs. The physiotherapist must ensure that the stairs are well lit, that there are adequate handrails and floor surfaces are non-slip.

Patients must also be instructed how to get in and out of bed safely, and in and out of chairs correctly. There must be a sufficient variety of chairs to suit all patients' individual needs, ideally brightly coloured and attractive and covered in a durable washable material for protection should accidents occur.

Patients with specific conditions such as hemiplegia, paraplegia, or an amputation, need a specialised individual rehabilitation routine and time must be spent building up confidence and trust between patient and physiotherapist. Where the patient's disability precludes him from walking, the physiotherapist must train him in the correct use of a wheelchair, specifically selected for him. Because of the patient's mental state instructions may have to be repeated many times before he learns what is required, but with patience and perseverance this can be achieved.

Chest conditions

Another area of importance is the treatment of chest conditions. Any loss of mobility is detrimental to respiratory function. On the whole patients do not like being given postural drainage and percussion and the treatment should not be given if the patient is confused and unable to co-operate. Many ruses have to be used to encourage the patient to cough. Although chest work is not easy, it can be essential and requires a great deal of skill and expertise. Patients generally will only tolerate so much, so to enable the treatment to be successful, the physiotherapist must work within the patient's toleration span. The maxim 'little and often' may be the only way.

Pressure sores

The physiotherapist has a valuable contribution to make towards the prevention and management of pressure areas by encouraging the patient's mobility, discouraging the use of restrictive-type chairs and by working closely with nursing staff to ensure relief of pressure and thus overall comfort of the patient by frequent and regular change of body position.

The effect of drugs

Physiotherapists must be aware of the side-effects caused by the various psychotropic drugs. The side-effects of particular importance are those which mimic the extra-pyramidal effects associated with Parkinson's disease (rigidity, tremor, muscle weakness, slowness of movement, mask-like expression, inability to keep still). Examples of drugs which can cause such symptoms are trifluoperazine (Stelazine) and chlorpromazine (Largactil). The physiotherapist has to determine whether the patient is exhibiting a true neurological condition or a drug-induced one.

These parkinsonian side-effects can be reduced by the administration of anti-parkinsonian drugs such as procyclidine (Kemadrin) or benzhexol (Artane).

Examples of psychotropic drugs which may cause photosensitivity and skin reactions are chlorpromazine (Largactil), chlordiazepoxide (Librium) and diazepam (Valium). This obviously has an influence on any treatment involving ultraviolet irradiation.

Group work

General exercise classes

Exercise classes are an ideal medium for helping to prevent contractures besides being an excellent therapy enabling patients to let go and enjoy themselves. Schemes of exercises must be chosen which ensure that all parts of the body are exercised. An extra dimension is added if music is used, which provides an ideal means of communication and can help relieve tensions and agitation. Patients should be consulted about the choice of music, if possible, so that a favourite tune can be played or another avoided if it has traumatic associations. This will help the patients to gain the maximum benefit and enjoyment from the sessions.

Classes are also an excellent means whereby the physiotherapist can monitor any potential problems.

Relaxation classes

Physiotherapists are skilled in the art of teaching relaxation and tension control, and relaxation techniques can be of tremendous value in the reduction of tension and stress. It must be remembered that not all elderly mentally ill patients are demented. Many suffer from depression, anxiety, personality disorders and other such conditions which can be greatly helped by relaxation. Many patients exhibit tension. Often they will sit for long periods in a tense position, i.e. shoulders hunched, arms adducted to the side, head, neck and elbows bent, hands tightly clenched, hips and knees flexed.

Very often such patients will be clutching some kind of comfort object, e.g. a hanky or tissue, which they are reluctant to release.

Relaxation can be given on an individual basis or in groups. Care must be taken over the timing of a session, as there are people whose tensions increase as the day progresses, while there are others who are more tense in the earlier part of the day. Whatever relaxation technique is chosen, some time must be given to an explanation of the techniques used, for if patients understand what is happening, more benefit will be gained from the treatment. At least an hour must be given for the session, and treatment must be reviewed frequently to see if it is still of benefit.

When setting goals and planning treatment programmes, the physiotherapist should try to take into account the patient's individual wishes even though these may be unrealistic. With time and persuasion, the patient may be enabled to accept more rational goals.

If there is no alternative to continuing hospital care and support, then all efforts must be directed towards enabling patients to retain some level of personal identity and social competence in an institutional setting.

Physiotherapists together with other staff involved, should ensure that patients' mobility and daily living skills are, where possible, maintained and improved and that patients are helped to participate in a range of activities that encourage choice and decision making and provide opportunities for social contact.

Advisory

Running parallel with the treatment of the patient is the advisory role of the physiotherapist. Because physiotherapists have specific skills and expertise they are particularly concerned with patients' physical problems and needs, and as a result should be prepared to advise their colleagues in other disciplines, relatives and other informal carers on the many aspects of the patient's physical care and management.

In addition, requests for information and advice on equipment such as hoists, wheelchairs, specialised beds and mattresses; on furniture, particularly suitably designed chairs; on the appropriate siting of handrails for lavatories or stairways; and on appropriate footwear, will come from a wide variety of sources. Among these will be hospital administration and supplies departments regarding feasibility and cost and choice of manufacturer.

Education

The role of the physiotherapist

'The primary role of the specialist physiotherapist member of the team is to ensure that the work of the physiotherapist is fully understood by nurses and others concerned' (HAS, 1982).

Care of the patient depends upon close co-operation of the multidisciplinary team. No individual professional group can work effectively without understanding the role of colleagues in other disciplines. This is a vital part of the framework of the working team. Multidisciplinary meetings and discussion provide excellent learning and teaching situations, with each professional contributing from the knowledge and experience of particular specialties. In reviewing individual patient's progress during regular case conferences for example, the physiotherapist's contribution to the overall therapeutic plan for each patient will be seen in context and more readily understood by all other disciplines concerned.

This understanding can be reinforced if there are opportunities for pre- and post-basic professional staff including doctors and nurses to spend time with the physiotherapist in her work either in the department, ward, day hospital or community.

Educational requirements for physiotherapists

The needs of elderly people with mental disorders require special attitudes and training by all staff concerned. Currently, physiotherapists acquire the greater part of this knowledge through 'on the job' experience. Greater exposure of students in training to centres of good practice, where psychiatric services for the elderly are progressive and innovatory, and more regular deployment of recently qualified physiotherapists within a district to work in psychiatry on a rotational basis, would do much to foster interest and develop understanding of this specialised field.

Attendance at seminars, study days and conferences and visits to specialised psychiatric services in other health districts to exchange information and discuss mutual problems and needs, will increase knowledge and help to maintain interest and enthusiasm.

Motivation and communication

Lack of motivation is one of the big problems faced by the physiotherapist. How does one motivate a patient to want to get better or to do something he does not want to do? Every situation is different.

Some patients are better motivated on an individual basis, while others respond to a group atmosphere. Whatever the case, the patient must see the physiotherapist as a person who cares about him and is interested in his well-being. This also goes a long way in helping his morale and self-esteem.

Motivation is dependent upon many factors. The personality of the physiotherapist is her most important therapeutic aid. Very often success of the treatment may be attributed to the physiotherapist's personality and ability to inspire confidence as much as to the treatments used.

The initial contact with the patient is crucial. He must be enabled to feel at ease, and in this way will develop confidence and trust in the physiotherapist. Establishing a relationship cannot be hurried and takes time regardless of other demands upon the physiotherapist. Any impatience will be transmitted to the patient and he will fail to respond. The physiotherapist must be prepared to sit and talk and to listen, and to answer questions honestly. Elderly patients are particularly sensitive to approval, disapproval and affection. The use of touch, taking the patient's hand, for example, can be a helpful way of developing communication.

Physiotherapists must know the patient's background, previous interests and psychiatric history, not only to avoid conversation which might be traumatic but also to understand the difficulties and problems experienced by the patient. In this context, personal questions may seem to the patient too direct and appear to be prying, so there has to be considerable sensitivity when acquiring information. Discussion with both community personnel with prior knowledge of the patient and visiting relatives or friends will help the physiotherapist to find the key to establishing contact and initiating some response. The physiotherapist's primary concern is the patient's welfare so patients have to be accepted on their terms and individual idiosyncrasies tolerated. On good days a great deal of progress can be made, while on bad days almost nothing. Moods can vary within seconds. The physiotherapist has to learn to be firm while remaining kind. A great deal of patience, tolerance and tact are needed in the treatment of the elderly mentally ill.

Time must be given for instructions to be followed. They may have to be repeated frequently, however simple, as memory may be poor. The therapist must always explain to the patient what is being done; even if they cannot communicate many patients do understand. Reassurance and encouragement must be given throughout all activity.

CONCLUSION

Physiotherapists can derive tremendous satisfaction and reward when working with elderly, mentally ill patients. This relatively new field of professional activity not only brings additional challenges for physiotherapists concerned, but the knowledge and skills acquired stimulate interest and deepen understanding. If attitudes are flexible so that activities can be co-ordinated with other disciplines involved, physiotherapy skills and expertise will be recognised and valued.

REFERENCES

Health Advisory Service (1982). *The Rising Tide: Developing Services for Mental Illness in Old Age*. NHS Health Advisory Service, Sutton, Surrey.

Pitt, B. (1976). *Psychogeriatrics. An Introduction to the Psychiatry of Old Age*. Churchill Livingstone, Edinburgh.

Chapter Ten

COMMUNITY PHYSIOTHERAPY FOR ELDERLY PEOPLE

by J. Stephenson MCSP

Community n. a body of people having common interests or environment; the public or people in general.

From this dictionary definition it would seem easy to place hospitals as part of the community. This has not always been the case, but reorganisation of the NHS in 1974, when hospital and community care were brought together under one umbrella, has enabled a growing number of health care professionals to cross the boundary between hospital and community, so that this artificial distinction is slowly beginning to disappear.

The introduction of the DHSS Health Note (1981) *Physiotherapy in the Community and Open Access to Physiotherapy Departments by General Practitioners* is leading to the development of closer liaison between hospital-based services and those of other care workers in the community in order that better services for patients and their relatives can be provided. Moreover, the DHSS emphasis on the need to prevent or minimise disability in order to enable elderly people to maintain independence at home and avoid the necessity of hospital admission has led to the growing availability of community-based physiotherapy services.

Although a number of community physiotherapy schemes have been established over the years as, for example, services for children in schools or the attachment of a physiotherapist to a GP pratice in a few places in the country (Partridge and Warren, 1977), it was only in the early 1970s that real development started. Since the mid-

1970s, community physiotherapy initiatives have accelerated rapidly. In 1978 there were 100 schemes nation-wide; by 1984 the figure had risen to 359.

ORGANISATION

Community physiotherapy schemes have developed in a number of ways according to geographic needs, available resources, including transport, and the priority given to their development by individual health authorities and district physiotherapists.

Community services may be provided by staff based in NHS establishments such as hospital physiotherapy departments, geriatric day hospitals, health centres or general practitioner premises. A number of health district staff may be deployed from home and this can be particularly useful where physiotherapists are unable to work fixed hours because of family responsibilities.

Where community schemes have been financed by statutory money, staff can be based in social services departments.

Domiciliary or community

'Various terms have been used to describe the practice of physiotherapy outside a hospital department' (Partridge and Warren, 1977). Those who call themselves 'domiciliary' physiotherapists, strictly speaking work in the patient's home (*domus* = home). The term 'community' is much broader in its definition, encompassing domiciliary physiotherapy plus a range of locations such as health centres, GP premises, schools, residential homes, day centres, church halls, etc.

The community and physiotherapy

Community physiotherapists work with all age-groups and in all areas ranging from ante-natal instruction to terminal care. They may be specialists in obstetrics or paediatrics or they may be generalists visiting patients of any age with any condition.

The major proportion of disabled adults living at home are over the age of 65 (Harris, 1971) and it follows, therefore, that the majority of patients on the general physiotherapists' case lists are likely to be elderly. Of patients referred for community physiotherapy in one health district 88 per cent were over the age of 60 (Ellman et al, 1982) and this is the trend generally.

THE COMMUNITY PHYSIOTHERAPIST AND ELDERLY PEOPLE

As already discussed (p. 57), only 6 per cent of retired people at any one time are in any form of institutional care, the remaining 94 per cent are living in the community the majority being independent, or managing with the help of relatives and friends.

Disabilities do, however, accumulate with age and conditions referred for physiotherapy cover a wide range, but with those that affect mobility and independence being referred most frequently. Cerebral vascular accident is the commonest cause of severe disability to be encountered in the community, although parkinsonism, defects of postural mechanism, musculoskeletal conditions and amputation of the lower limb following peripheral vascular disease are among other diagnoses involved.

Physiotherapists working with elderly people in the community have both a therapeutic and supportive role with regard not only to the patient and his family but to other carers involved, both voluntary and professional. The support is educational in nature and may be provided on both a formal and informal basis.

In assessing problems of management, identifying goals and planning appropriate action, much informal teaching is involved for both patient and relative. More formal education is provided in, for example, lifting or handling techniques for professional staff concerned (p. 127).

Following referral and identification of problems the physiotherapist must be prepared to select appropriate patients for community physiotherapy or to refer to other agencies.

Aims of community physiotherapy

The overall aim which is shared by all community workers is to prevent or postpone the necessity for admission to hospital of vulnerable people and to facilitate earlier discharge for those who are in hospital.

The more specific aim of the community physiotherapist is to provide a holistic approach to the rehabilitative needs of the patient in order to restore and maintain maximum functional ability and to prevent or retard deterioration.

Assessment, treatment planning and advice

Community physiotherapy is generally regarded as an assessment and advisory service, with the emphasis on prevention and self-help rather than on long-term treatment.

1. Assessment must be made of *all* factors affecting the patient's physical capabilities – his home environment (and problems encountered here will be far removed from those found in the hospital gymnasium); his mental state; his motivation; his carers' attitude, as well as his physical condition.

   Many of these factors are difficult to record objectively but it is essential that all such contributing influences are identified if accurate assessment is to be made.

2. Realistic goals must be established and a programme of management planned, taking into account the aspirations and lifestyle of the patient and the demands made on other carers involved.

   The emphasis of treatment will be on improving functional ability in order to restore quality of life rather than on isolated regimes of exercise.

3. If the advice offered to both patient and carer is to be acceptable and useful, it must not only be practical and responsive to individual needs, but also comprehensive and persuasive.

   Motivation must be encouraged, confidence boosted and the effectiveness of the treatment plan, in terms of the patient's increasing ability to understand and use what he has learned (compliance) must be measured and recorded. Equipment needs generally to be simple and kept to a minimum. Improvisation should be second nature to the community physiotherapist. For example, packets of frozen peas make useful ice packs, and a pile of stacked newspapers can be used to supplement pillows when carrying out postural drainage.

   Depending upon the service provided and the physiotherapist's mode of transport, equipment can vary from a saw and a stock of ferrules, or a range of walking aids, to sophisticated electro-medical instruments in some cases. Nursing aids, or aids for daily living activities are provided by the relevant statutory agencies and the ease with which they can be ordered by the physiotherapist will depend on local arrangements.

THE COMMUNITY PHYSIOTHERAPIST AND THE DISTRICT PHYSIOTHERAPY SERVICE

The DHSS recommend that adult community physiotherapy schemes should be managed as part of the total district physiotherapy service.

Regular personal contact with colleagues working in all hospital clinical specialties in the health district, including psychiatry, is a necessity, not only to ensure that the community physiotherapist knows the range of resources and facilities available but also that hospital colleagues understand her role and refer appropriately. It is also important that community physiotherapists do not become

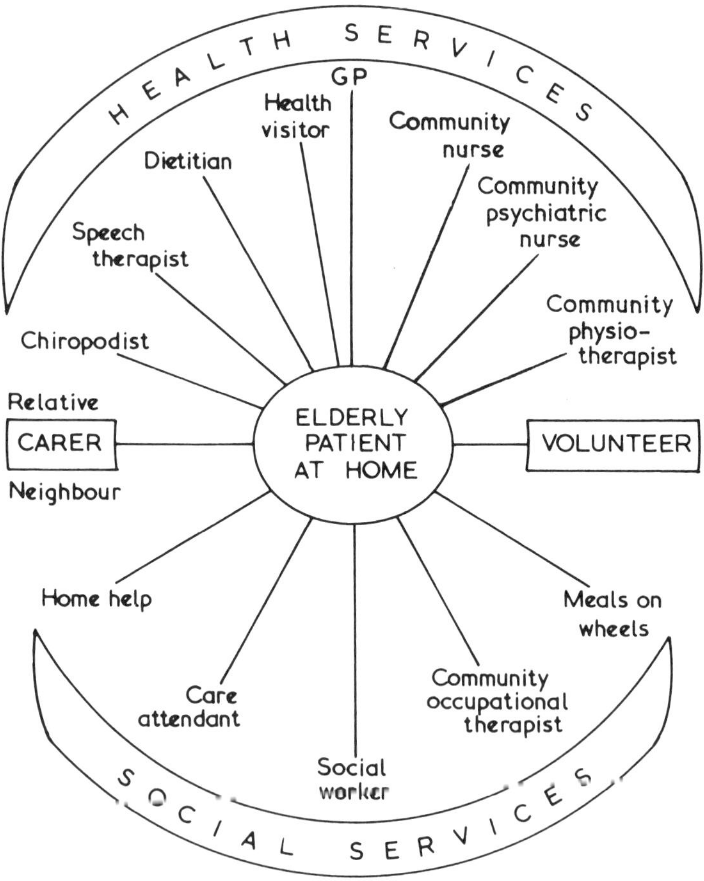

Fig. 10/1 The elderly patient in the community

professionally isolated, but are accepted as an integral part of the district physiotherapy service.

THE COMMUNITY PHYSIOTHERAPIST AND THE MULTIDISCIPLINARY TEAM

Two-way interchange is essential between the physiotherapist and the wide network of multidisciplinary personnel working in the community (Fig. 10/1). Both insight into individual roles (Chapters 4 and 5) and co-operation through regular communication at case conferences and primary care team meetings ensure continuity of patient care as each discipline's contribution to the total management plan is known to each member concerned.

Following assessment the physiotherapist must be prepared, when necessary, to enlist additional assistance. Examples of this might be consultation with the occupational therapist; day hospital intervention; the referral to a local stroke group of a hemiplegic patient or encouraging a patient and his family to contact one of the self-help groups associated with his particular disability, such as the Parkinson's Disease Society.

Working with community personnel

General practitioners refer their patients for community physiotherapy assessment either directly or through a member of the primary care team. If the referral is received from someone other than those, e.g. social services, the physiotherapist must report her involvement following an initial assessment, particularly if the assessment indicates the need for physiotherapy treatment.

Community nurse

Because patients with long-term problems are visited regularly and frequently by community nurses, an opportunity is provided to monitor closely any changes in individual physical states. Discussion with the community physiotherapist may indicate the need for physiotherapy assessment. Moreover, a joint visit to the patient's home with the nurse will enable the physiotherapist to reinforce lifting and handling techniques or perhaps confirm the nurse's opinion that the doctor's advice should be sought.

Health visitor

Where both a community physiotherapist and a health visitor make regular visits to the patient at home, to assess his continuing ability to maintain health and physical independence, close communication is essential so that each can alert the other at an early stage if any deterioration in his capabilities has occurred. In this way duplication is prevented.

Community psychiatric nurse

Where elderly people are both mentally and physically disabled, the co-operation and combined expertise of the community psychiatric nurse and physiotherapist can provide practical help and guidance for the family so that more effective management can be achieved.

Social worker

The physiotherapist's assessment of the patient's ability to continue managing independently at home is an essential contribution to the social worker's overall evaluation of the patient's needs.

Community occupational therapist

Close working relationships with occupational therapy colleagues will ensure that the patient's functional abilities are assessed comprehensively. Where the patient presents with mobility problems and the physiotherapist is first involved, the decision will be made following initial assessment to refer to the occupational therapist where appropriate.

Similarly, the occupational therapist may seek the physiotherapist's opinion where it is thought that a person's potential for improvement in range of normal movement, may obviate the use of an aid to daily living.

Speech therapist

Speech therapy advice and treatment can be provided for elderly people with speech and language disturbance either in their own homes or in the local health centre or day hospital. It is important that the community physiotherapist and the district speech therapy staff co-operate closely, so that continuity of management can be established for patients requiring help from both disciplines.

THE COMMUNITY PHYSIOTHERAPIST AND EDUCATION

The patient and informal carers

The patient's education is an integral part of the overall plan of management. Recording the procedure by the problem orientated method allows for retrospective evaluation of the effectiveness of the physiotherapy teaching.

When elderly patients with mobility problems live alone without the help of relatives or other informal carers, activities to improve functional ability will be taught by the community physiotherapist on a one-to-one basis. When carers are available, however, the physiotherapist can involve them in the reablement programme by teaching them how to give effective help and encouragement. In such cases the patient may be described as receiving 'indirect physiotherapy'.

Formal caring staff

Caring personnel such as home helps, residential and day care staff, nursing auxiliaries and family aides, work with frail elderly and disabled people in their own homes, in residential accommodation or in day centres and other day-care establishments. For all these staff it is essential, both in terms of their ability to help the elderly client and in terms of their own job satisfaction, that they receive good in-service training (Age Concern, 1983).

The principle underlying all such teaching by community physiotherapists is that caring staff should understand the need to encourage and enable elderly people with mobility problems to maintain independence and to avoid activities that foster dependence. At the same time, by learning to use correct methods of lifting and handling, carers can diminish fatigue and risk of back injury.

THE ROLE OF THE COMMUNITY PHYSIOTHERAPIST IN THE PATIENT'S HOME

Providing physiotherapy for a patient in his own home rather than in hospital necessitates a different approach. The physiotherapist needs to remember at all times that she is a guest in the home and attitudes must be adjusted accordingly. Sensitivity to family relationships and individual lifestyles and an awareness of the additional demands that will be made on already overburdened relatives, possibly themselves elderly, are important aspects to be taken into account when carrying out treatment programmes.

There may be a number of caring personnel involved with the patient at home and this can be confusing for him, so it is important that the community physiotherapist makes clear and acceptable arrangements for the initial visit.

The first appointment may be made by telephone and a mutually convenient time for the visit agreed. Alternatively, the patient can be contacted by post and a date and time proposed. Details of the source of the referral for physiotherapy, the reason for it and the name of the patient's general practitioner should be included in the correspondence. Time should be given for the patient to reply in case the proposed date is unsuitable.

On arrival at the patient's home, the physiotherapist should introduce herself to the patient and his family, referring to her previous telephone call or letter. A visiting card with a contact number may be given to the patient if appropriate. Some physiotherapists find that wearing uniform may overcome problems of identification, particularly if the patient has some previous experience of hospital physiotherapy. Others find that a more comfortable relationship can be established if normal everyday clothing is worn.

By allowing the patient to lead the way into his living room opportunity is provided for unobtrusive observation of his posture and gait and the suitability of his walking aid and footwear. The design and stability of the chair which he is accustomed to use and the ease with which he is able to sit down or rise from it are important factors to be noted. Stock should also be taken at this time of any potential hazards to safety in the home, such as floor space cluttered with furniture, loose mats on the floor, a trailing light flex or inadequate lighting on steps or stairs.

All such information will help to alert the physiotherapist to the realities of the patient's overall problems and needs.

During initial discussion, which may include the relatives or concerned friend or neighbour, further general surveillance can be made of the patient's sitting posture, appearance and state of health. In time the conversation can be gradually steered towards a more structured verbal examination.

A brief medical history must be noted and this will be particularly concerned with the events contributing to the patient's presenting problems, his drug regime and the number of other disciplines who may be involved with his support.

The physiotherapist will need to probe gently for all relevant information. It may be that difficulties will be uncovered which will require the intervention of other agencies. Alternatively, further enquiry may reveal that the patient's perception of his main problem differs from that given in the original referral. For example, a history of recent falls may have been the reason for the request for physiotherapy, whereas on questioning it becomes clear that failing eyesight is the root of the patient's problem – a factor with which, he admits, he has not liked to bother his busy doctor.

The physiotherapist's assessment of each patient should be a continuing process, and throughout the period of treatment she should be alert to any new problems or changes in individual circumstances that may arise.

If there is a specific musculo-skeletal or neurological problem, a thorough subjective and objective examination must be made of such factors as range of movement, muscle strength and tone, and of sensory perception. The patient's own comments regarding any dysfunction must always be noted.

For people with severe mobility problems, assessment of functional activities, such as the ability to move in bed, to transfer from bed to chair, and to lavatory or commode, must involve members of the family or other carers concerned. They will require practical demonstration and guidance on methods of lifting and handling and on the importance of correct positioning to minimise spasticity for those who have suffered a stroke and on the avoidance of excessive dependence on the sound side of the body.

Falls in the home are a common occurrence among very elderly people and will require careful assessment by the community physiotherapist. Failing vision and hazards in the home previously mentioned, are among risk factors associated with falls. Others include hypotension, the side-effects of certain drugs or impairment in balance or in mobility. Advising on safety factors in the home, improving the patient's balance and walking ability, and teaching him ways of getting up from the floor independently or with appropriate help are important aspects of the physiotherapist's role in the home.

New methods of management should be introduced gradually over a series of visits so that patient and carer are not overburdened with instructions and feelings of confusion and inadequacy can be avoided. Carers' abilities can be continuously monitored and appropriate reinforcement given where needed, so that confidence is gradually built up. They must be helped to understand how much to expect the particular patient to achieve and gentle guidance provided in instances where the carer tends to be over protective.

Planning the patient's living environment to meet his physical capabilities, so that he is enabled to function with maximum ability is an essential part of the treatment programme. Uncluttered floor space to facilitate walking or wheelchair mobility, the appropriate positioning of furniture and the adequate adjustment in the height of bed, chair and lavatory to aid ease of transfer are essential requirements if independent living is to be restored or management made easier for the carer.

However, alterations of this nature may need to be approached with tact and diplomacy. Re-arrangement of a bedroom or living room, removal of loose rugs from the floor or the replacement of a favourite 'easy' chair by one more suitably designed to promote independence, will not always be accepted readily by an elderly person somewhat set in his ways or by a houseproud daughter in whose house the patient may be living.

Major re-arrangements which may involve alterations to the patient's previous lifestyle will need to be thought through with care. For example, while the decision to bring the patient's bed downstairs may overcome the problem of climbing stairs, it may overlook the fact that if the carer continues to sleep upstairs, difficulties are created for the patient who requires help during the night.

In seeking to meet the multiple needs of patients at home the physiotherapist must recognise when to enlist the help of other professional personnel. For example, she will need to work closely with the community occupational therapist in assessing the patient's physical environment, involving such factors as the optimum location of grab or stair rails or the appropriate width of doorways for the wheelchair patient. If a need is identified for day hospital attendance, co-operation and consultation with the general practitioner will be required. Alternatively, if the patient is living alone and is socially isolated, then the physiotherapist may contact the local social services department to discuss the possibility of regular day centre attendance to provide support.

Establishing liaison and successful working relationships with personnel in both statutory and voluntary agencies is frequently time consuming and far from easy, but it is essential if continuity of patient care and management is to be effectively maintained.

THE ROLE OF THE COMMUNITY PHYSIOTHERAPIST IN RESIDENTIAL CARE

Old people's homes contain a higher proportion of residents well over the age of 75, many of whom grow increasingly dependent as their stay in the home increases. Because care staff frequently lack basic knowledge of the principles of human movement, such frail and disabled residents are given inappropriate help which tends to undermine mobility and independence.

The educational role of the community physiotherapist in residential homes can be summarised as follows:

1. To assess and advise individual residents with physical disability and give appropriate guidance to care staff involved.
2. To participate in training programmes for staff and to teach the principles involved in lifting and handling techniques and in providing appropriate help so that independence and mobility can be encouraged.
3. In the absence of regular occupational therapy attendance at the home, to advise on environmental needs and suitable furniture, particularly the problems of restrictive and inappropriate seating (HAS, 1982).
4. To conduct exercise groups and to teach residents about the value of exercise in health maintenance.

Professional staff

Participation in formal training and up-dating courses for professional community personnel, sharing knowledge with physiotherapy colleagues working in hospital and providing opportunities for physiotherapy students either on community placement or in schools of physiotherapy to learn about the skills required, are all components of the community physiotherapist's role in education.

THE COMMUNITY PHYSIOTHERAPIST AND HEALTH EDUCATION

A community physiotherapist has a considerable role to play in providing health education. Through her everyday work with elderly patients the emphasis is on the prevention of further disability and in maintaining function and a healthier existence and this philosophy will be transmitted to other carers involved.

Teaching correct body mechanics, posture and movement to community staff to prevent back injury, and talks to pre-and post-retirement groups on the value of exercise in the maintenance of a healthy later life are some of the ways in which the physiotherapist can be involved in health education and prophylaxis.

CONCLUSION

The development of community physiotherapy has particular advantages for elderly people. It obviates the need for out-patient physiotherapy and thus avoids the distress, frustration and socially disruptive effects of ambulance transport, caused by long waits and tedious journeys. Learning to improve physical function and mobility in the familiar home environment engenders confidence not only in the patient but in his carers also.

The nature of the work demands from the physiotherapists concerned, maturity, a wide experience and a range of skills, not least being the ability to provide specialist advice and guidance to all those who are helping with the patient's management and support.

Not only does community physiotherapy provide a valuable alternative to the more traditional hospital-based service and frequently at lower cost (Frazer, 1980) but, to the physiotherapist involved any difficulties encountered are well outweighed by the rewarding experience of helping to improve the quality of life for many elderly people.

REFERENCES

Age Concern England (1983). *Training Helpers in Caring for the Elderly*. Age Concern, Mitcham, Surrey.

DHSS (1981). Health Note: *Physiotherapy in the Community and Open Access to Physiotherapy Departments for General Practitioners*. Available from: DHSS Store – Health Publications Unit, No 2 Site, Manchester Road, Heywood, Lancashire DL10 2PZ.

Ellman, R. et al (1982). Making physiotherapy more accessible. *Physiotherapy*, **68**, 9, 291–3.

Frazer, F. W. (1980). Domiciliary physiotherapy – cost and benefit. *Physiotherapy*, **66**, 1, 2–7.

Harris, A. I. (1971). *Handicapped and Impaired in Great Britain*. HMSO, London.

Health Advisory Service (1982). *The Rising Tide. Developing Services for Mental Illness in Old Age*. NHS Health Advisory Service, Sutton, Surrey.

Partridge, C. J. and Warren, M. D. (1977). *Physiotherapy in the Community*. Health Services Research Unit, University of Kent, Canterbury.

Chapter Eleven

INCONTINENCE

by D. Mandelstam MCSP, DipSocSc

There is a real need for a positive and informed approach to the care of the incontinent patient especially where nothing has been done to ameliorate the problem. Incontinence is a symptom, not a disease, and when understood it can be treated, alleviated or managed. While it is customarily associated with elderly people, it does in fact occur at any age. However, there are many precipitating factors in older people which make them more vulnerable.

Understanding the cause of the incontinence as well as the form it takes has an essential bearing on how to deal with it. The therapist helping the patient to achieve personal independence has to consider excretory function. Independence in this respect is not only important to self-esteem, but it can govern the kind of life the patient can lead and the quality of that life. Elderly people, whether living at home or in some form of institutional care, are frequently already in a dependent situation due to frailty or disability, and if incontinence is added to this their dependence on those who care for them is inevitably increased.

There is no other symptom which causes such distress to patients and carers alike. This distress unfortunately is sometimes accompanied by hostility on the part of the carer. Excreta deposited in unsuitable places produces interminable work of washing and cleaning, as well as understandable distaste.

MECHANISM OF MICTURITION

The bladder is a contractile hollow organ acting as a reservoir for urine, and when a certain pressure is reached the contents are expelled through the urethra. In dynamic terms micturition occurs when the bladder pressure (intravesical) exceeds that in the urethra. In recent years the practice of urodynamics has involved the study of the function and dysfunction of the lower urinary tract (bladder and urethra). Methods of investigation have evolved, including pressure measurements, enabling disorders to be diagnosed with some accuracy (Feneley, 1980).

The closure of the bladder outlet influences the pressure and is dependent on a number of anatomical and physiological features. These are: the intra-urethral pressure regulated by smooth and striated muscle; the anatomical relation of the urethra to the base of the bladder (bladder neck); and the pelvic floor muscles and fascia. The mechanism of neurological control includes the pelvic nerves of the 2nd, 3rd and 4th sacral segments of the spinal cord with the associated reflex arc and the relevant area of the brain (cerebral cortex) (Fig. 11/1).

Continence is the ability to empty the bladder at will at a suitable time and in a suitable place. This skill, which consists of the ability to inhibit bladder contractions and to postpone voiding remains throughout life unless the control mechanisms are diminished. Incontinence may therefore result from organic changes in the bladder, affecting its capacity as a reservoir, the urethra and its supports, and the nervous control as described.

Organic causes

There are many physical causes and some degree of medical assessment is essential, but observation of the habits and needs of the patient, as well as the degree of leakage occurring, can point to the underlying condition. Medical or surgical treatment may be required but often the need is for good nursing management, especially with elderly people.

For simplicity the causes and types of incontinence can be divided into those affecting the lower urinary tract and those relating to the nervous system (Tables 11/1 and 11/2).

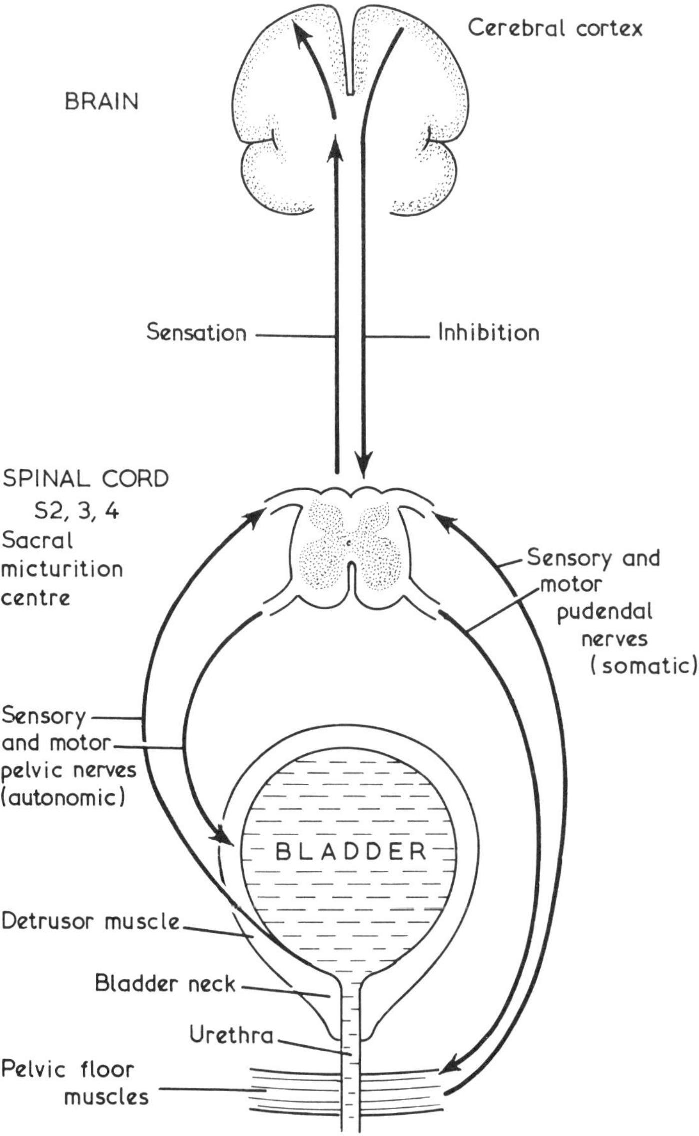

Fig. 11/1 The neurological pathways involved in micturition

Table 11/1 Local Organic Incontinence

Causes	*Type*
Irritation of bladder, e.g. cystitis, stone, tumour, and over-activity of the 'irritable' or 'unstable' bladder	Urgency and frequency, which may lead to uncontrollable voiding of bladder contents
Partial obstruction of outlet flow, e.g. prostatic enlargement, uterine fibroids, faecal impaction (very common in older people)	Retention with overflow incontinence. The bladder becomes over-distended so that the intravesical pressure remains constantly higher than the closing pressure and leakage is continuous, in dribbles or spurts
Mechanical trauma in the female. This may arise following childbirth due to overstretching of fascia and pelvic muscles, resulting in an inadequate closure mechanism. Women who have not borne children may sometimes be affected	Stress incontinence: a small leakage on exertion. A large leakage may occur if on exertion an involuntary bladder contraction is set off (unstable bladder)
Mechanical trauma in the male. This may occur after injury to the urethra and sphincter mechanisms, from fractures of the pelvis or after prostatectomy	Stress incontinence

Table 11/2 Central Nervous System Incontinence

Causes	*Type*
Damage to the peripheral nerves, e.g. operative trauma, diabetic neuropathy, tabes dorsalis	Retention with overflow incontinence; the bladder becomes grossly distended as awareness of fullness is lost, with dribbling leakage
Lesions of the spinal cord, spinal injury, spina bifida	Automatic reflex emptying of contents of the bladder with absence of sensation
Lesions of the brain, e.g. cerebrovascular accidents	(a) awareness of need but inability to exercise control (b) loss of conscious ability to inhibit voiding of bladder contents
Loss of consciousness, e.g. coma, epileptic fit	Automatic emptying of the bladder

Other causes

Incontinence may also occur indirectly due to emotional factors such as bereavement, anxiety or other emotional states which influence morale or motivation. For instance, institutional care of an entirely custodial kind can in itself induce states of apathy and indifference (Newman, 1962). He describes the experience of prisoners of war in the Korean campaign where confinement to an unfamiliar environment, conformation to an inflexible routine and deprivation of normal relationships caused prisoners to become indifferent to their surroundings, depressed, dishevelled and incontinent.

Diminished mobility or dexterity which impedes independence in getting to the lavatory and in managing there unaided is a frequent cause of incontinence. Attention in the home to such environmental factors as improving access to toilet facilities; the provision of a downstairs lavatory; the use of an appropriate aid such as a raised lavatory seat or suitably placed handrails may be all that is needed to improve personal function and alleviate problems of incontinence. In hospitals and residential homes, similar principles will apply. Toilet facilities, designed for wheelchair use and to accommodate people with walking frames, should be sufficiently numerous to ensure that elderly people are within 10 metres (30 feet) distance of a lavatory at all times. An adequate number of commodes need to be available, particularly at night time, and beds of suitable height provided to facilitate use of commode or lavatory.

Whether at home or in institutional care, some people are enabled to maintain independence by using a small personal urinal (for women the Sub-a-Seal is an example) if placed within easy reach.

Nursing management

For people in institutional accommodation, insufficient awareness of individual needs in relation to emptying the bladder may lead to 'accidents'. If, for example, bladder control is precarious, help will be needed quickly and may arrive too late. The effect of this on an elderly person endeavouring to hold on to some shreds of self-respect can be the final humiliation.

When staff are organised on a patient- rather than a task-centred basis, individual variations in continence control can be identified and recorded and action taken accordingly. Such an approach sees continence as a goal to be promoted rather than incontinence as a disease to be treated (*BMJ*, 1978).

The general management of the patient will be the responsibility of the nurse, involving the initial assessment including charting, toilet regimes and/or the use of equipment. However, the therapist requires detailed information about the various practices so that she may co-operate in any plan for the patient. As a member of a multidisciplinary team she will be working with others to find the most effective individual approach, bearing in mind the following points:

1. Has the pattern of micturition been monitored and charted and what does it show? Is the toileting round adequate for the patient's needs? If there is no pattern and the patient is unaware of wanting to pass urine, has a different regime been implemented? A rigid toileting scheme can establish regular emptying (Browne, 1978; Clay, 1980).
2. Can the patient indicate her need particularly if aphasic? Would a bell or card saying 'Toilet Please' be of help?
3. The mechanics of using a urinal or lavatory may have to be re-taught if, after a stroke, the patient suffers from motor or sensory disturbance, particularly problems of apraxia or visual agnosia.
4. Could access to the lavatory be made easier and quicker?
5. Would the use of a commode be more suitable? Is it the right

height for comfort and ease of transfer from bed or chair?

6. Has the patient adequate privacy? This is of fundamental importance.
7. Can clothes be quickly and easily managed?
8. If the patient has a form of intractable incontinence and requires equipment, has there been an assessment of what is most suitable? There is a variety of protective pads and pants available for both sexes. Appliances for men, to date, are more ergonomic than anything available for women.

Recent developments

In the last few years there have been a number of significant advances in incontinence care. There are several incontinence clinics and an increasing number of incontinence nurse advisers. This has led to the development of new techniques and expertise both investigatory and practical. For example intermittent non-sterile self-catheterisation, a technique developed initially for patients with spinal injury, is now being tried in patients with multiple sclerosis and in elderly patients with a reflex bladder. In this way someone without neurological control over the bladder can empty it mechanically, swiftly and conveniently, so doing away with the need to use pads or devices.

It will be evident to the therapist that she, as well as the nurse, needs to keep herself informed about new management techniques and the available range of all forms of aids and equipment. If she is not fortunate enough to have access to an incontinence nurse adviser, other sources of information are given on page 142.

Specific therapy relating to the pelvic floor

In appropriate cases re-training the pelvic floor muscles alleviates the symptoms of stress incontinence. Theoretically there is no age limit to training but the patient must be able to understand and remember the teaching, and the therapist must verify by digital examination that the correct muscles are being used. Asking the patient to stop and start the flow of urine is a useful way of developing muscle awareness and furthermore of making the patient conscious of a means of control. The following simple instructions, addressed to the patient, will help to develop control:

Sit or stand. Without tensing the muscles of your legs, buttocks or abdomen, imagine that you are trying to control the passing of a stool by tightening the ring of muscle around the back passage. This will help you to become aware of the back part of the pelvic floor.

When you are passing urine, try to stop the flow, then re-start it. Do this every time you empty your bladder. Gradually you will become aware of the front muscles of the pelvic floor.

Working from the back to the front tighten the muscles while counting to four slowly, then release them.

Do this four times, once an hour or as often as you can for a period of three months. The exercise can be done anywhere – sitting or standing, while watching television or waiting for a bus.

This simple prophylactic technique should be taught as a routine exercise to women of any age-group.

Bladder discipline
In some patients with urgency and frequency (unstable bladder) the habits of the bladder can be altered. The patient is asked to void by the clock rather than from any natural desire and to increase the interval between emptyings. Pelvic floor contractions can be used to reinforce this effort when asking the patient to hold on and not to void in between the allotted times. This can be reinforced by the patient sitting on a sandbag or a hard surface.

FAECAL INCONTINENCE

Faecal incontinence, although it occurs less frequently than urinary incontinence, is more distressing to patients, relatives and staff. The action of the bowel, however, can be more successfully controlled than that of the bladder. Causes may be medical conditions, trauma to the ano-rectal muscle producing faulty function, or brain lesions and dementia.

On the other hand, in elderly and immobile people the most common cause of incontinence, both urinary and faecal, is faecal impaction. This can result from neglect of call to stool, diminished awareness of the feeling of a full rectum, feeble peristaltic movement, incomplete evacuation and impairment of the mechanism of defaecation. Faeces accumulating in the rectum or colon become dehydrated and compacted, leading to the passage of more fluid stools seeping past the impacted mass (spurious diarrhoea). Attention to the normal bowel habit of the individual patient is particularly important in the prevention of this problem.

Although the majority of people expect to pass a motion every day, bowel frequency can in fact range from three actions a week to three a day. The picture of normal defaecation in an individual, however, depends on information not only about frequency but volume and consistency of stool. All these factors require detailed observation on admission to hospital, where change of routine, diet and fluid intake and a period of immobility can upset the patient and lead to constipation. The therapist is not directly involved in bowel management, but she will no doubt be aware of the mechanical and psychological difficulties arising from the use of bedpans and commodes, the lack of privacy in wards, and diminished activity. Patients naturally prefer to use the lavatory, even if they have to be wheeled there. They also like to be able to lock the door, and to find lavatory paper within reach. The therapist, by being alert to these needs, can ensure that suitable practical measures are taken.

CONCLUSION

Incontinence is a complex but common problem, causing much distress to sufferers and supporters. Identification of the cause followed by appropriate treatment and/or management in each individual situation can lead to dramatic improvement.

Attitudes, however, take time to change. Traditionally, incontinence has been accepted as part of the expectations for older people – an inevitable consequence of ageing and therefore irreversible and untreatable.

Because of the physiotherapist's particular knowledge and expertise, she can do much to help. As a professional concerned with the practice of rehabilitation, she cannot ignore the implications of incontinence in relation to the the independence and well-being of the patient.

A positive and informed approach to the subject can do a great deal to combat attitudes of defeatism and will help to improve facilities and, hopefully, lead to a more adequate range of resources.

Where appropriate, specific therapy to the muscles of the pelvic floor can be particularly effective in the field of prevention and in the treatment of patients with stress incontinence or an unstable bladder.

Where disability is the major cause of incontinence, the physiotherapist, in co-operation with others involved, will be concerned in increasing physical function and mobility, in providing aids to greater independence and in helping to improve and adapt lavatory facilities to meet individual needs.

REFERENCES

Browne, B. (1978). *Management for Incontinence.* Age Concern England, Surrey.

Clay, E. C. (1980). Rehabilitative nursing. In *Incontinence and its Management*, (ed Mandelstam, D.). Croom Helm Ltd, London.

Editorial (1978). Incontinence. *British Medical Journal*, **1605**, 61.

Feneley, R. C. L. (1980). Normal micturition and its control. In *Incontinence and Its Management*, (ed Mandelstam, D.). Croom Helm Ltd, London.

Newman, J. L. (1962). Old folk in wet beds. *British Medical Journal*, 1824–7.

INFORMATION

The Incontinence Advisory Service of the Disabled Living Foundation provides advice and information to professionals as well those affected by incontinence. There is also a training and education service.

The Association of Continence Advisors is a multidisciplinary group of health care professionals with a special interest in the promotion of continence and the management of incontinence.

Further information about these services may be obtained from: The Disabled Living Foundation, 380–384 Harrow Road, London W9 2HU

Chapter Twelve

DRESSING NEEDS FOR ELDERLY PEOPLE

by P. Turnbull MCSP, DipPE

Recovery or even improvement in a person's physical or mental state cannot easily be achieved, even by skilled treatment, unless that person is motivated to reach the desired goal. Personal appearance is closely allied to state of mind; to be well groomed and well dressed can do much to restore or maintain morale and self-respect, providing incentive to participate in a normal social life.

To dress oneself is essential for independent living and even those who need assistance experience some sense of achievement if they can accomplish even a small degree of self-help. The inability to manage clothing when going to the lavatory, or using a hand-held urinal, can be a stumbling block to independence and can often lead to incontinence.

Physiotherapists know the handicaps associated with disease and need to be aware of the relationship of these to clothing and dressing when assessing patients either in hospital, at home or in other residential accommodation. Close co-operation with others involved with the patient, professional and non-professional, not to mention discussion with the patient himself, should ensure that dressing problems do not hamper rehabilitation. Physiotherapists can actively help in many instances, for example showing how best to relieve muscle spasm which interferes with a patient's ability to dress himself or be dressed by others.

Most elderly people, even those handicapped by disability, can wear normal up-to-date clothes if the garments selected are easy to put on and take off, can be managed without difficulty when using the lavatory and, especially for those who have to sit for long periods, are comfortable to wear.

Other individual needs may have to be considered, such as clothes to camouflage figure faults, to keep cold limbs warm or to cope with dribbling. Particular problems are created for those who have to wear awkward body or limb appliances, use crutches or propel a wheelchair.

Sometimes a new method of dressing will need to be adopted, perhaps making use of a dressing aid; for example, stroke patients and others with unilateral disability must learn to put affected arms and legs into sleeves and pants first (last out when undressing). It may be that a simple adaptation to a garment will help, such as substituting elastic for the ribbon shoulder straps of underwear. Frequently a handicapped person will have discovered, by trial and error, the best way of getting in and out of clothes. Therapists need to explain to helpers how the patient's disability will affect his capacity to dress and undress unaided. Often by simulating such handicaps themselves, helpers can experiment with new dressing methods before trying them out with patients.

Old people need sufficient time to dress themselves, and to be helped when it is necessary, to prevent exhaustion and frustration leading to cessation of effort with accompanying demoralisation and apathy. Warmth and privacy are essential. Physiotherapists can show how best to position the old person so that he will be safe and comfortable when dressing. They should remind helpers that any walking or dressing aids, body appliances or prostheses, wheelchairs or footstools which may be required must be to hand and furniture arranged to provide safe support where needed.

A confused person will find it helpful if clothing is laid out in order of dressing and in such a way that the garments can be picked up and put on without re-adjustment. Hold-up stockings, pop socks and some men's socks which have no heel shaping may be easier to position on feet. Patient guidance will be needed over weeks of constant repetitive practice if some measure of independent dressing is to be achieved.

Dressing can be made difficult in many ways as the result of disease. Movement may be painful, limited in range and of reduced strength and endurance. Other presenting problems might include, for example, disorders of sensory perception, alterations in muscle tone, disturbance of postural control and inco-ordination or weakness of limbs. Visual impairment is another factor that will often need to be taken into account.

FEATURES WHICH WILL HELP TO IMPROVE GARMENTS' SUITABILITY TO MEET INDIVIDUAL NEEDS (Fig. 12/1(1–18))

Comfortable fit

Loose comfortable fit can be achieved by choosing a fabric with 'give', such as a knit, or a woven fabric can be used on the bias, and by selecting a garment design which assures fullness where needed, which has deep roomy armholes and trouser legs with sufficient width (1). Partially or fully elasticated, or otherwise adjustable waistbands can also be helpful. A-line dresses and skirts can be put on more easily, are more comfortable when the wearer sits and easier to pull up out of the way when going to the lavatory.

Accessible openings

Ample accessible openings to garments are important. The type of opening will depend largely upon the way the individual finds it easiest to dress; this may be by putting the garment over the head or the feet or, if there is a full front opening, by putting the garment on like a coat.

Clothing which is put on over the head can have a smaller opening, without fastenings, such as a sweater, if it is roomy and the fabric has plenty of stretch. However, larger front openings, preferably to below waist level, make it easier to dress in many instances. A long back opening may be more suitable if shoulders are very stiff and painful but the wearer will probably need to use a zip aid (2).

Capes and ponchos can be thrown over the shoulders avoiding the difficulties of a garment with sleeves. Wrap-around skirts will have similar advantages.

Fastenings

Easily managed, accessible fastenings can be crucial to the achievement of independent dressing but difficult garment fastenings can be modified.

Velcro is a valuable fastening medium which needs only a touch to close. It will be less efficient if the hooks get clogged with fluff and *the fastening should always be closed before laundering*. Where the strain against the fastening is considerable at least 5cm (2in) contact is needed, but using long lengths, which are difficult to align, should be avoided.

1.

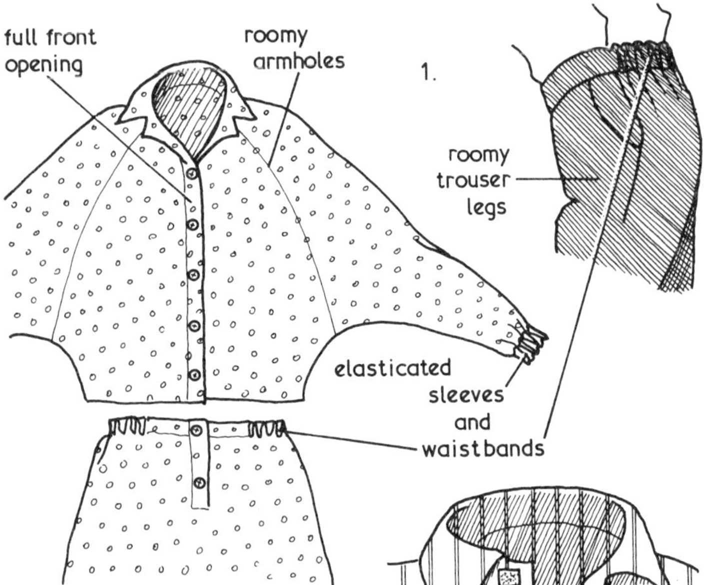
full front opening
roomy armholes
roomy trouser legs
elasticated sleeves and waistbands

2.

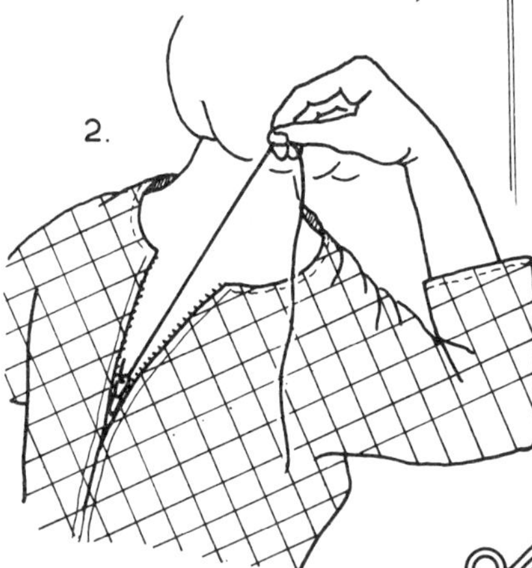

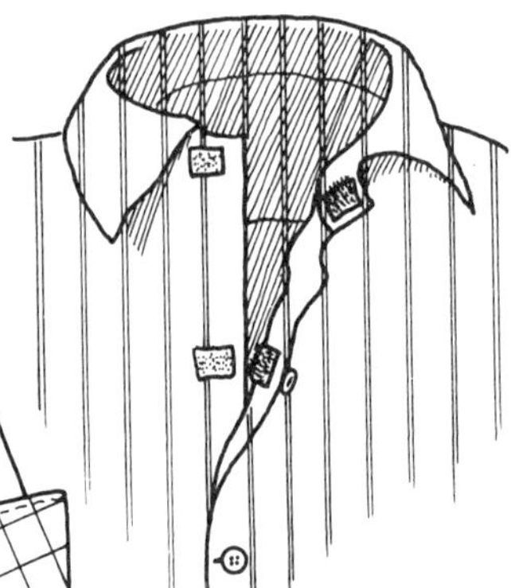

3.

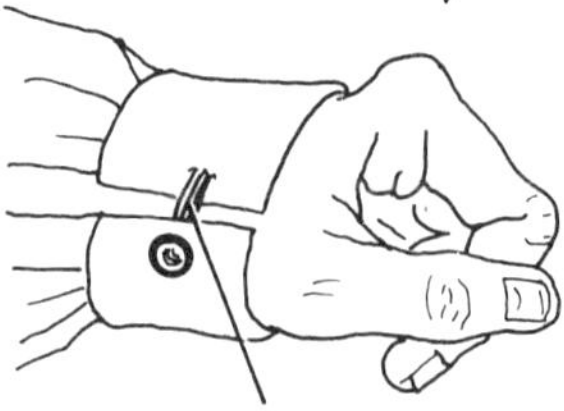
elastic thread

4

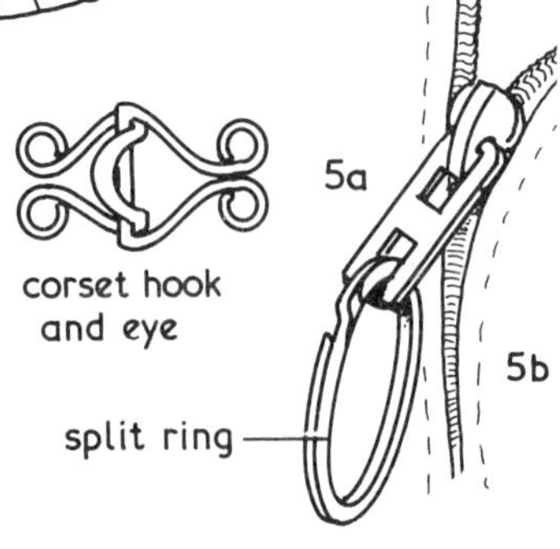
corset hook and eye
5a
5b
split ring

If small buttons are sewn on top of buttonholes, Velcro underneath makes an easy to manage fastening and the appearance of the garment is unchanged (3). Large buttons and buttonholes may be easier to close than small ones but are not always appropriate on a garment. Difficult cuff buttons can be sewn on with elastic thread so that the hand can be pushed through without unfastening (4).

Corset hooks and eyes can replace the smaller type often used on foundation garments; the eye curves away from the body and is much easier to hook (5a). A large split-ring attached to a zip puller can also help (5b).

By far the most difficult fastenings to manage, especially if only one hand is available, or the grip is weak, are those where there are opposing pulls. Examples of these are bra, corset and suspender belt fastenings, trouser or skirt waistbands and suspenders. Velcro used together with a strap and D, or rectangular, ring can pull the two sides of an opening together so that any further fastenings can be completed without difficulty (6). Sliding bar buckle and hook-fasteners (Kempner fasteners) can be used similarly (7), and are often used to fasten surgical corsets. Both these fastenings need to be positioned so that the pulls is towards the stronger hand.

Suspenders can be fastened to stockings more easily, even with the use of only one hand, if they are detached from the garment to which they belong. The free end of the suspenders can then be re-attached to the garment using any of the methods shown (8). Alternatively, a simple elastic suspender belt can be made; this is fastened around the body after the suspenders have been fastened to the stockings (9).

Additional factors

Garments which have to be pulled over the hips when the wearer is unable to stand, or over the feet when it is difficult to bend down, pose particular problems.

Some people may find it easier to dress on a bed and the physiotherapist can teach them how to 'bridge' so that garments can be pulled up or down over the hips (10). Alternatively, if they are taught to roll from side to side the clothing can be eased over the hips a little

Fig. 12/1 Dressing aids and adaptations. 1. Achieving a loose comfortable fit. 2. Zip dressing aid. 3. Button fastening replaced by Velcro. 4. Stretch cuff fastening. 5a. Corset hook and eye. 5b. Easily grasped zip pull.

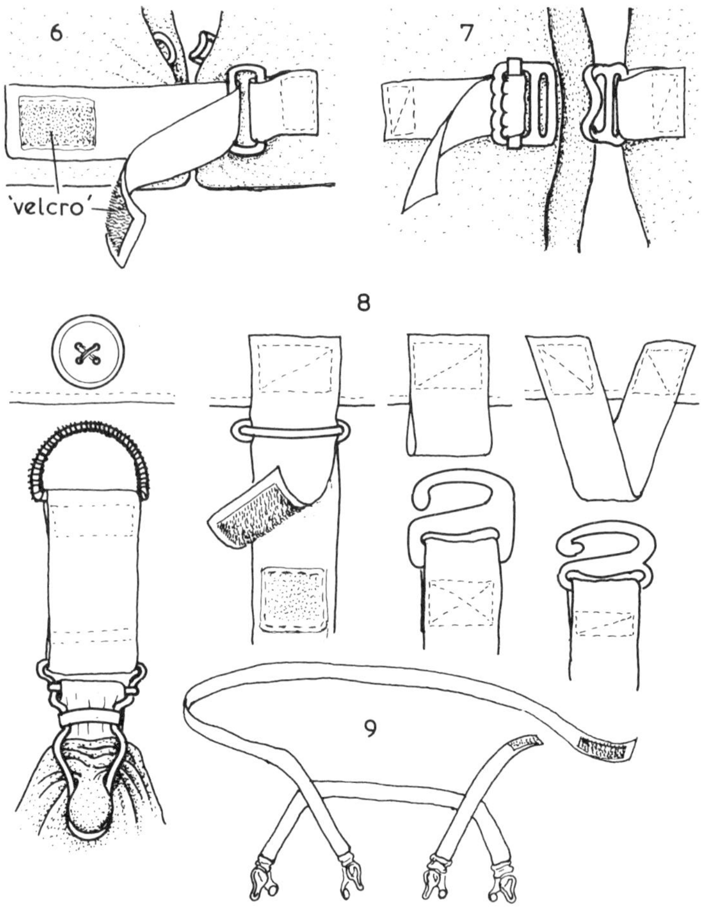

Fig. 12/1 *cont.* 6. Velcro strap and ring fastening. 7. Kempner fastener. 8. Methods of fastening detached suspenders. 9. Do-it-yourself suspender belt.

at a time. Similar methods can be practised sitting on a chair, rocking from buttock to buttock.

If clothing has been carefully chosen, it can be got out of the way quite quickly with practice when going to the lavatory. It may sometimes be necessary to add a side-opening, or openings, if undoing

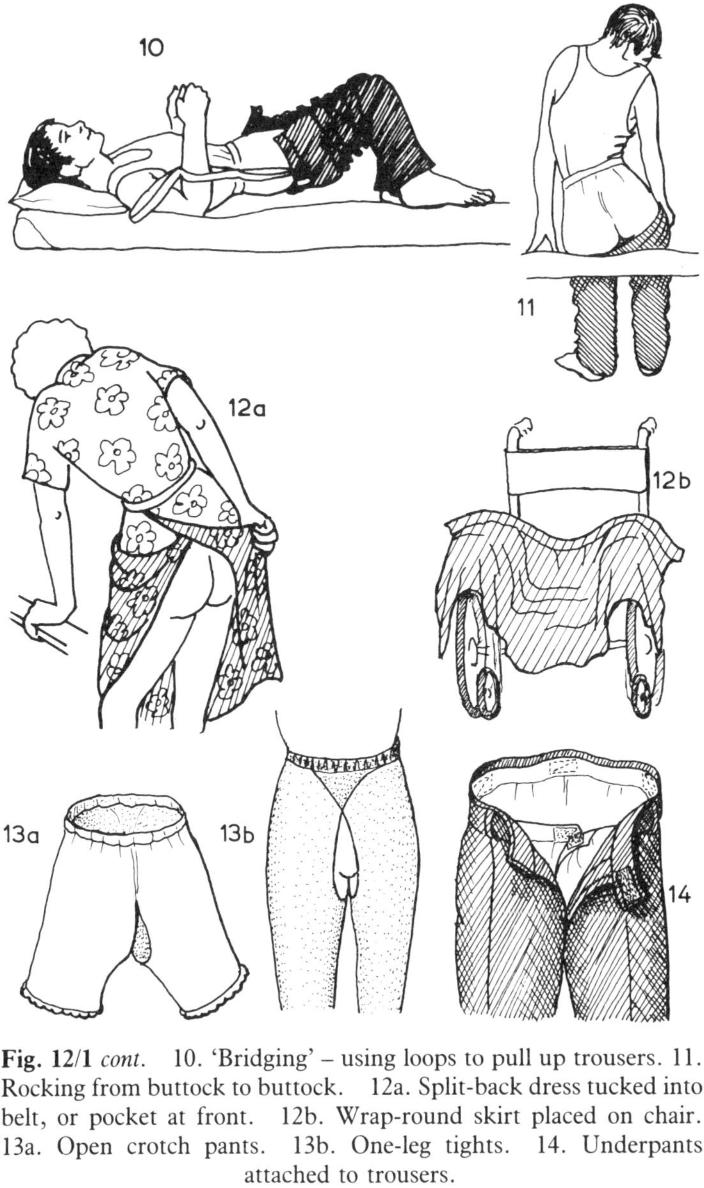

Fig. 12/1 *cont.* 10. 'Bridging' – using loops to pull up trousers. 11. Rocking from buttock to buttock. 12a. Split-back dress tucked into belt, or pocket at front. 12b. Wrap-round skirt placed on chair. 13a. Open crotch pants. 13b. One-leg tights. 14. Underpants attached to trousers.

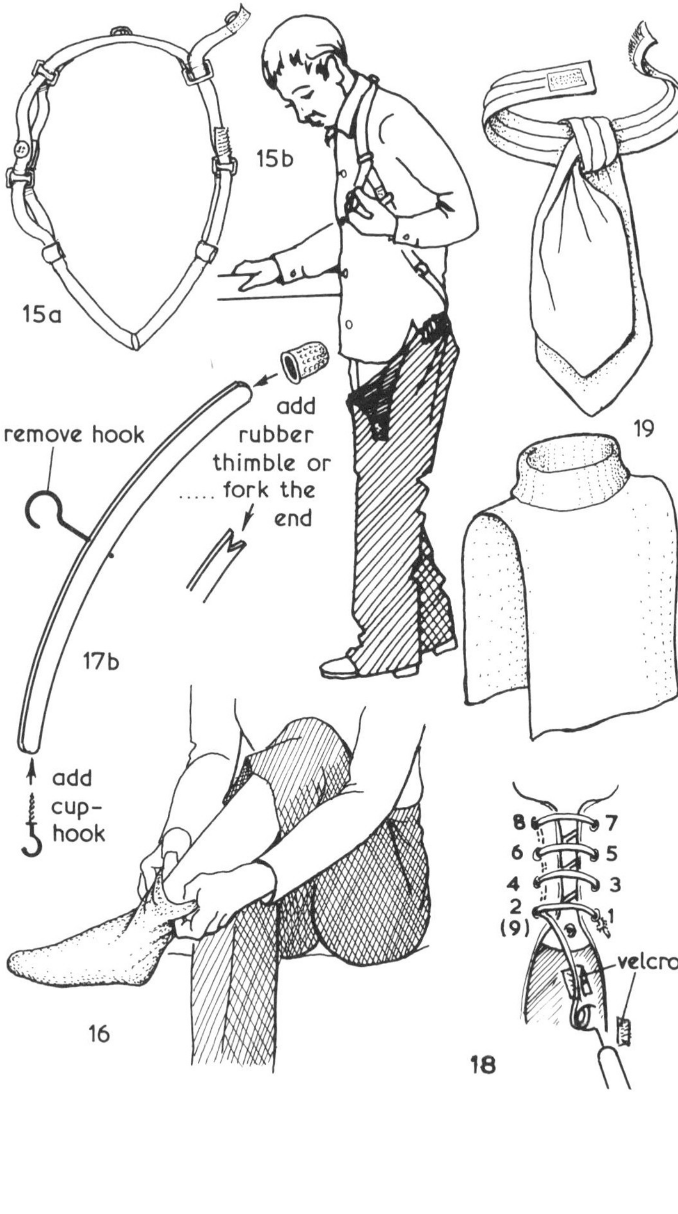
15a
15b
remove hook
add rubber thimble or ..... fork the end
17b
add cup-hook
19
16
8 7
6 5
4 3
2 1
(9)
velcro
18

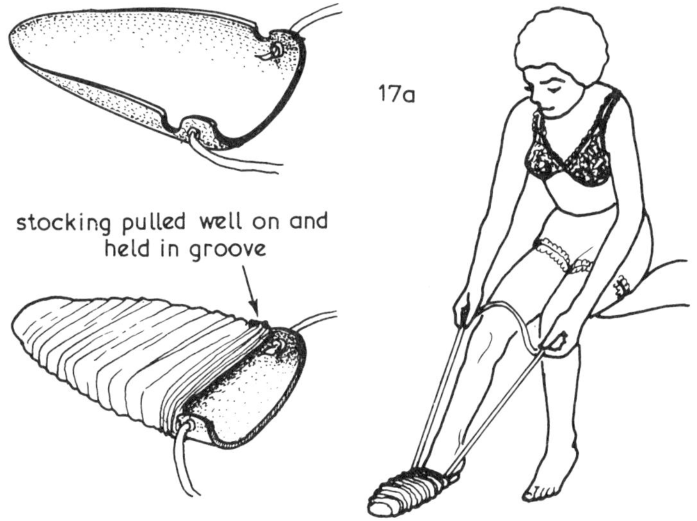

Fig. 12/1 *cont.* 15a. 'Edgware' braces. 15b. Lowering trousers using 'Edgware' braces. 16. Easier to reach the foot. 17a. Stocking gutter with stocking pulled over the foot. 17b. Home-made dressing stick. 18. Shoe lace fastening using a dressing stick. 19. Back-fastening cravat and polo-necked dickey.

the front fly alone of tight fitting trousers is not enough. A dress or skirt may be particularly awkward to keep out of the way if the wearer's hands are not free to hold the garments when standing or transferring.

Garments that separate or wrap over at the back are useful (12a). Dresses, skirts, slips and nightwear of this type can be put on over the head or wrapped around the waist without the person needing to stand. The two sides of the back can quickly be pulled to the front and tucked into a belt or pockets and kept out of the way without holding. A skirt which wraps over at the front can be left behind on a wheelchair when the user transfers to the lavatory (12b).

Sometimes when the need to micturate is very urgent the dressing methods described cannot be managed sufficiently quickly and it may be helpful to wear pants that can be pulled to one side, or apart at the crotch. Loose french pants, combinations, and special open crotch pants (13a) are all possibilities as are open crotch tights or single leg tights (13b).

Men's underpants can be adapted to open at the front waist, attached to their trousers with Velcro dabs (14), and thereafter the two garments can be pulled up and down as one, halving time and effort. Men who need to use a urinary bottle when sitting find 'Edgware' trousers, which open right into the crotch and have a high back 'rise', convenient to wear. 'Edgware' braces (15a) designed so that trousers can be lowered (15b) and retained without the need to remove jacket, sweater, and so on, can sometimes be helpful to a stroke patient who has insufficient balance to bend down and pick up the trousers if they fall to the ground.

When bending down is difficult, other ways must be tried to get garments and shoes over feet, and a therapist with knowledge of the patient's limitations can advise. People find strange ways of coping – one elderly woman, with adducted hips and no hip flexion, was able to balance on one leg, bending the other back at the knee and somehow lasso the free foot with shoe suspended on the end of her walking stick! Many old people may find it easiest to sit and cross one leg over the other knee (16) while others like to use a footstool or the side of a low bed.

Dressing aids can be useful, such as long-handled shoe horns, stocking gutters (17a), loops sewn on garments (10), dressing sticks (17b) and other aids which help to extend reach. If a shoe is laced as shown and a hole made in the top of the tongue, a hooked dressing stick can be used to hold up the tongue when inserting the foot and to fasten the laces (18). Alternatively elastic laces can convert a shoe into a slip-on (tongue should be sewn down one side).

Hospital patients and people in residential accommodation should have little difficulty in keeping warm but at home it can be another matter. Warmth will depend on the insulation provided by the still air trapped in the fabric weave, knit and surface finish, in the garment construction, and in between garments and between the garment and skin. The greater the surface area of the body covered, including the head, the warmer the person will be. Wool which shrinks on washing can lose valuable air spaces. However, these days alternative lightweight clothing is not difficult to obtain.

CLOTHING FLAMMABILITY

Open fires in the home, cooking over a gas burner, or heavy cigarette smoking can present hazards for elderly people and their supporters if the combustible nature of certain clothing materials is not appreciated. These hazards may be exacerbated if the particular garment involved is loose and flowing in style, with full rather than well-fitting sleeves.

FOOTWEAR

Unfortunately, an item of clothing seen all too frequently is the sloppy slipper, with trodden-down heel, held on the foot solely by means of the wearer's shuffling gait. Not only is the wearer at risk from falls but the poor walking pattern which develops, with little exercise of the calf muscles, does little to help disperse the postural oedema so often present when an old person sits for long periods of time. A shoe which fits firmly over the instep and at the heel, which should be low and broad, is much more satisfactory. If the old person cannot be persuaded away from slippers then the bootee type, with front fastening, at least allows normal walking. If these slippers have a centre front and back seam they can easily be opened and adapted should the feet become very swollen or need heavy bandaging.

Some quite attractive ready-to-wear shoes are being made by orthopaedic footwear firms and semi-made-to-measure shoes, inexpensive in comparison to the NHS made-to-measure variety, are also available. These shoes can have extra depth as well as width and go some way to accommodate some of the very difficult feet found in adulthood.

A PERSONALISED CLOTHING SERVICE

In order to encourage maintenance of personal identity in the artificial world of hospital, elderly patients should be enabled to wear their own or personally allotted clothes. The degrading practice of sharing communal hospital-supplied clothing can destroy individuality and self-esteem.

Choice of suitable clothing, together with any necessary adaptations, is based on accurate assessment of need. However, such efforts will be fruitless unless the facilities provided by a personalised clothing service are available in order that each patient's stock of garments, once selected, can be adequately stored, laundered and maintained for his or her own exclusive use.

Having attained a personal clothing service, it is up to all staff to help keep clothing clean and attractive. Physiotherapists can make sure that patients have chairs and tables of the right height and are sitting sufficiently close at meal times to avoid food spills on clothing. Any that do occur should be fielded by a napkin, well tucked in, not an undignified bib. Bibs should also be avoided if there is a dribble problem, although some protection for clothes will probably be necessary. With a little imagination something more acceptable can be devised such as the illustrated back-fastening cravat or polo-necked dickey (19) (see p. 150). Physiotherapy treatment to try to control the dribbling can sometimes be effective.

Incontinence, its causes and management, is discussed in Chapter 11. However, protection of clothing by the intelligent use of special pants and pads, need not preclude training for continence and will do much to preserve the dignity and self-respect of individual sufferers from this distressing condition.

FURTHER READING

The following books are published by, and available from, the DLF (Sales) Limited, Book House, 45 East Hill, London SW18 2QZ.

Dean, F. (1982). *Clothing Needs of the Elderly Person.*
Hughes, J. (1983). *Footwear and Footcare for Adults.*
Macartney, P. (1973). *Clothes Sense for Handicapped Adults of All Ages.*
Ruston, R. (1982). *Dressing for Disabled People.*
Turnbull, P. (1982). *A Guide to the Introduction of a Personalised Clothing Service.*

In addition *Information Lists*, particularly *Clothing* (No. 13) and *Footwear* (No. 14), which are annually updated, are available from the Information Service of the Disabled Living Foundation, 380–384 Harrow Road, London W9 2HU.

Information papers on various clothing topics are available from the Clothing Adviser, DLF Clothing Advisory Service, 380–384 Harrow Road, London W9 2HU.

Clothing and Dressing for Adults: Equipment for the Disabled. This book is produced by Mary Marlborough Lodge, Nuffield Orthopaedic

Centre, Headington, Oxford OX3 7LD. It is updated approximately every four years (5th edition 1981).

ACKNOWLEDGEMENT

The illustrations in this chapter have been adapted from illustrations in the Disabled Living Foundation publications, *Incontinence*, *Clothes Sense for Handicapped Adults of all Ages* and *Dressing for Disabled People*.

FINAL THOUGHTS

Our ageing population is not a single-time phenomenon, it has long-range perspectives which have profound implications for all of us both as self-interested citizens concerned about the society in which we hope to live in old age and also as professional health workers. Most older people live in the community. Little is known of the well-functioning majority and they make but 'fleeting contact with hospital services' (Muir Gray, 1984).

Even when ill and disabled, people want to continue living in their own homes retaining personal autonomy and some measure of self-dependence. But for them and their supporters the odds against them can be incredibly high. The recent tendency to cut down on time in hospital, frequently puts extra burdens on families and other informal carers. The growing disenchantment with institutional care and the general acceptance of the therapeutic importance of preserving individual lifestyles, personal identity and family and neighbourly links, reinforce central Government policy on the general shift towards community care. Increasing expectations of disabled people themselves for the right to services that enhance dignity and self-respect, the pressures on carers and the dangers of institutionalisation are all important factors that need to be taken into account when planning use of scarce resources.

But as we have seen, the provision of health and social services support for people in their own homes is remarkably incoherent. Remedial therapy too 'has developed as a highly specialised service' (Helander, 1976) whose growth cannot begin to match demand.

Although the majority of disabled people live in the community, the majority of physiotherapists in the National Health Service are hospital based. Currently 'only 23 out of 167 district health authorities can meet the demands for community physiotherapy services' (Williams, 1984), and not all services are concerned with elderly people.

The need for physiotherapy skills to be more available to the public generally so that intervention at an earlier stage of disability can be initiated and health promotion and preventive work encouraged is urgent. Much lip service is paid to the concept of health promotion and the prevention of avoidable disability. Physiotherapists have an important role to play in stressing the value of exercise, in encouraging older people to be active and self-reliant and not to accept disability as a necessary accompaniment to ageing.

Closer collaboration between health and social services and a more flexible use of staff across hospital and community boundaries would facilitate more effective deployment of scarce personnel. Initiatives such as the use of task forces or multidisciplinary peripatetic teams based on day hospitals, health centres or group general practices are being developed in some parts of the country. Patients referred to hospital can be visited at home by a member of the team, so that continuity of support and management for the patient concerned can be maintained throughout the period of his treatment whether home or hospital based. Another innovatory idea is the concept of the 'stroke' flying squad which can organise early intervention for a stroke sufferer and provide support for the family involved.

Working with disabled people and their supporters through domiciliary care staff and the primary care team, physiotherapists can do much to encourage self-care and prevent physical deterioration.

> The effectiveness of a minority group such as physiotherapists should be measured not only by what they can achieve as isolated clinicians but by what others can do as constant attenders.
>
> Having identified the strategy, our role is to work with others in order that they may feel informed, confident and able. We must share our skills and our knowledge if we are to have a definite and lasting effect (Rushfirth, 1983).

For physiotherapists clearly a re-orientation away from traditional hospital-based practice to the community would do much to meet current needs. Moreover, the more selective use of costly hospital resources and greater utilisation of the patient's home environment would eliminate the need for ambulance transport involving, as it does for many elderly patients, fatigue, anxiety and disruption of social life.

Substituting the patient's home for an out-patient physiotherapy department also allows physiotherapists greater freedom from routine and palliative treatment situations and enables them to have a more effective, dynamic and responsible role. Meaningful explanation of the disease processes to patient and family and skilled help with the management of disability foster self-care and confidence and avoid the dangers of perpetuating dependency implicit in hospital attendance.

Although such socialisation of our physiotherapy practice by the growing emphasis on its teaching and enabling role creates some paradoxes for our science-based and physically-orientated profession, this does not diminish the need to develop more sophisticated, technological methods for treatment measurement, teaching and research.

In the final count, however, our professional services must be responsive to current need. Faced with the multiple physical, mental and social problems of elderly people we have to be prepared not only to accept a new concept of ourselves as initiators, teachers and advisers, to acknowledge that our skills frequently lie in knowing what to do rather than actually doing it, but also to 'see beyond the health needs of the individual patient to the wider health needs of the whole community' (Abel-Smith, 1976).

REFERENCES

Abel-Smith, B. (1976). *Value for Money in Health Services*. Heinemann Educational Books Limited, London.

Gray, J. A. M. (1984). Care in the community. *Physiotherapy*, **70**, 4, 143.

Helander, E. (1976). *World Strategy for Disability Prevention and Rehabilitation*. World Health Organisation, Geneva.

Rushfirth, S. (1983). We must learn to share our skills. *Therapy Weekly*, December 8.

Williams, J. (1984). Address at Spring Seminar of Community Health Council Secretaries. *Remedial Therapist*, 7, 17.

FURTHER READING

In addition to the books and papers listed at the end of each chapter, the following represents a further select list of reading.

Adams, G. (1981). *Essentials of Geriatric Medicine*, 2nd edition. Oxford University Press, Oxford.

Agate, J. (1979). *Taking Care of Old People at Home*. George Allen and Unwin, London.

Arie, T. (ed) (1981). *Health Care of the Elderly*. Croom Helm Ltd, London.

Bergmann, K. (1972). *The Aged – Their Understanding and Care*. Stellar Press, Hatfield, Herts.

Bromley, D. B. (1974). *The Psychology of Human Ageing*. Penguin Books, Harmondsworth.

Caird, F. I. and Judge, T. G. (1979). *Assessment of the Elderly Patient*, 2nd edition. Pitman Medical, London.

Carver, V. and Liddiard, P. (eds) (1978). *An Ageing Population. A Reader and Sourcebook*. Hodder and Stoughton, London.

Centre for Policy on Ageing (1981). *Keeping the Elderly Moving in Old People's Homes*. CPA, London.

Cochrane, G. M. (1982). Hidden resources for rehabilitation and care of the disabled. *Journal of the Royal Society of Medicine*, **75**, February.

Corr, C. A. and Corr, D. M. (1983). *Hospice Care: Principles and Practice*. Faber and Faber, London.

Frazer, F. W. (ed) (1982). *Rehabilitation Within the Community*. Faber and Faber, London.

Gray, J. A. M. (1983). *Better Health in Retirement*. Age Concern England.

Gray, J. A. M. and McKenzie, H. (1980). *Take Care of Your Elderly Relative*. George Allen and Unwin, London and Beaconsfield Publishers, Beaconsfield.

Hall, D. A. (1978). The ageing process. Two theories explained. *Modern Geriatrics*, 66–7.

Hodkinson, H. M. (1981). *An Outline of Geriatrics*, 2nd edition. Academic Press, London.

Holden, U. P. (1984). *Thinking it Through*. The Winslow Press.

Hooker, S. (1981). *Caring for Elderly People*. Routledge and Kegan Paul, London.

Institute of Consumer Ergonomics (1983). *Selecting Easy Chairs for Elderly and Disabled People*. From 75 Swingbridge Road, Loughborough, Leics.

Jackson, O. (ed) (1983). *Physical Therapy of the Geriatric Patient*. Churchill Livingstone, Edinburgh.

Judge, T. G. and Caird, F. I. (1978). *Drug Treatment of the Elderly Patient*. Pitman Medical, London.

Lubbock, G. (ed) (1983). *Stroke Care: An Interdisciplinary Approach*. Faber and Faber, London.

Mandelstam, D. (1977). *Incontinence*. Published for the Disabled Living Foundation by Heinemann Health Books, London.

Mitchell, L. (1984). *Healthy Living over 55. The Getting-on Guide*. John Murray, London and Central Independent Television, Birmingham.

Mitchell, L. (1977). *Simple Relaxation*. John Murray, London.

Pitt, B. (1976). *Psycho-Geriatrics. An Introduction to the Psychiatry of Old Age*. Churchill Livingstone, Edinburgh.

Sitting and seating (1984). *Physiotherapy*, **70**, 2, 40–83.

Ransome, H. E. (1980). The role of the physiotherapist in homes for the elderly. *Physiotherapy*, **66**, 1, 324–31.

Twining, C. and Chapman, J. (1983). The clinical psychologist's input into the geriatric team. *Geriatric Medicine*, **1**, 41–6.

Whitehead, J. M. (1974). *Psychiatric Disorders in Old Age*. Harvey Miller and Metcalf, Aylesbury.

The following handbooks are updated yearly.

Your Rights for Pensioners (1984). Age Concern England.

Disability Rights Handbook (1984). The Disability Alliance Educational and Research Association, 25 Denmark Street, London WC2H 8NJ.

USEFUL ADDRESSES

This is a random selection of the many organisations from whom additional help and information may be obtained. The local Citizens Advice Bureaux will have additional lists of local organisations.

Age Concern England
Bernard Sunley House
60 Pitcairn Road
Mitcham, Surrey CR4 3LL

British Geriatrics Association
1 St Andrew's Place (From mid-1985)
London NW1 4LE

British Red Cross Society
9 Grosvenor Crescent
London SW1X 7EJ

Centre for Policy on Ageing
Nuffield Lodge, Regents Park
London NW1 4RS

Chest, Heart and Stroke Association
Tavistock House North
Tavistock Square
London WC1H 9JE

Counsel and Care for the Elderly
131 Middlesex Street
London E1 7JF

Crossroads Care Attendant Schemes
94a Coton Road
Rugby CV21 4LN

Cruse
Cruse House
126 Sheen Road
Richmond, Surrey TW9 1UR

Disabled Living Foundation
380–384 Harrow Road
London W9 2HU

Disablement Income Group
Attlee House, 28 Commercial Street
London E1 6LR

Help the Aged
32 Dover Street
London W1A 2AP

The Kings Fund Centre
126 Albert Street
London NW1 7NF

Mary Marlborough Lodge
Nuffield Orthopaedic Centre
Oxford OX3 7LD

National Health Service Health Advisory Service (HAS)
Sutherland House, 29/37 Brighton Road
Sutton, Surrey SM2 5AM

Rehabilitation Engineering Movement Advisory Panels (REMAP)
Thames House North, Millbank
London SW1P 4QG

Women's Royal Voluntary Service
Head Office: 17 Old Park Lane
London W1Y 4AJ

SPECIFIC INTEREST GROUPS

The following Specific Interest Groups of the Chartered Society of Physiotherapy may be contacted by letter to the secretary of the relevant group addressed c/o The Chartered Society of Physiotherapy, 14 Bedford Row, London WC1R 4ED.

The Association of Chartered Physiotherapists in Geriatric Medicine
The Association of Chartered Physiotherapists in Psychiatry
The Association of Community Physiotherapists
The Association of Chartered Physiotherapists with a Special Interest in Neurology

INDEX